The Comprehensive Guide to COLORECTAL CANCER

Dr Robinson M. Smith

Copyright © 2024 Dr Robinson M. Smith

All Rights Reserved. No part of this book may be reproduced, scanned, or distributed in any printed or electronic form without permission. Please do not participate in or encourage piracy of copyrighted materials in violation of the author's rights. Purchase only authorized editions.

Disclaimer

The information provided here is for educational purposes only and not intended as a substitute for professional diagnosis, treatment, or care. Consult your physician or qualified healthcare provider for any medical concerns. Please note, this resource is not a remedy but intended for management purposes only. Individual responses to treatment may vary, and personalized medical guidance is essential for proper diagnosis, treatment, and management of health conditions.

Table of content

Introduction...5
    Welcome and Acknowledgments....................7
    About This Guide...9
    How to Use This Book...................................... 11
Chapter 1: Understanding Colorectal Cancer..........14
    What is Colorectal Cancer?............................. 14
    How Does Colorectal Cancer Develop?................. 15
    Causes and Risk Factors.................................15
    Types of Colorectal Cancer............................. 19
    Signs and Symptoms......................................22
    Diagnostic Tests and Screening...................... 25
Chapter 2: Treatment Options...................................28
    Overview of Treatment Approaches....................... 28
    Surgery.. 30
    Chemotherapy... 32
    Radiation Therapy... 35
    Targeted Therapy..38
    Immunotherapy...40
    Clinical Trials and Experimental Treatments.......... 43
Chapter 3: Coping with Diagnosis...........................47
    Emotional Impact of Diagnosis....................... 47
    Communicating with Loved Ones.................. 49
    Finding Support.. 51
    Managing Fear and Anxiety............................55
    Making Treatment Decisions.......................... 57

Chapter 4: Navigating Treatment............................... 61
    Preparing for Treatment..61
    Managing Side Effects..65
    Nutrition and Diet During Treatment....................... 68
    Exercise and Physical Activity................................ 72
    Integrative Therapies and Complementary Medicine. 75

Chapter 5: Recovery and Rehabilitation...................79
    Post-Treatment Care.. 79
    Monitoring for Recurrence....................................... 82
    Rehabilitation and Physical Therapy...................... 85
    Coping with Long-Term Side Effects........................88
    Returning to Work and Normal Activities................ 92

Chapter 6: Living Well with Colorectal Cancer........ 95
    Lifestyle Changes for Prevention and Management... 95
    Nutritional Guidelines for Survivorship....................98
    Exercise and Physical Activity Recommendations..... 101
    Stress Management and Mental Well-Being........ 104
    Sexual Health and Intimacy.................................. 107

Chapter 7: Resources and Support..........................111
    Finding Reliable Information and Resources........ 111
    Financial Assistance and Insurance..................... 114
    Legal Rights and Advocacy................................... 118
    Additional Support Services..................................121

Chapter 8: Stories of Hope and Inspiration............125
    Personal Stories from Survivors and Caregivers.. 125
    Overcoming Challenges and Finding Strength..... 128

Messages of Hope and Encouragement.............. 132
Conclusion.. **135**
Appendices.. **137**
    Glossary of Terms.. 137
    List of Helpful Websites and Organizations.......... 140
    Index.. 143

Introduction

Let's be honest, life can throw some serious curveballs. A colorectal cancer diagnosis might feel like the biggest, baddest one yet. Maybe you're wondering, "Why me?" or feeling lost in a sea of medical jargon. Trust me, you're not alone.

But here's the thing: you've got a fight in you. You've faced challenges before, and you'll face this one too. This guide is your teammate, stepping into the batter's box with you. We'll break down the complexities of colorectal cancer in a way that makes sense, no fancy doctor talk here.

Think of this as your personal playbook for the game ahead. We'll explore everything from prevention strategies to the latest treatment options, giving you the knowledge to make informed decisions. We'll also show you how to fuel your body with the right "food plays" and keep your spirit high with exercise tips.

This journey might have unexpected twists, but with the right support system, you can hit a home run. We'll connect you with a community of people who understand, offering encouragement and sharing their own experiences.

So, take a deep breath, adjust your cap, and get ready to step up to the plate. This guide is here to help you turn this diagnosis into an opportunity to learn, grow, and ultimately, live a life that's as vibrant as ever. Let's rewrite the script and make this a story of strength, resilience, and a whole lot of living!

Welcome and Acknowledgments

Welcome to "The Comprehensive Guide to Colorectal Cancer." If you're reading this book, it means you or someone you care about has been diagnosed with colorectal cancer. Or maybe you want to acquire more knowledge about Colorectal Cancer. We know this is a difficult time, and we understand that you're likely feeling overwhelmed with questions and uncertainties. This book is designed to be your guide, offering information, support, and practical advice as you navigate this journey.

Our goal is to provide you with clear, easy-to-understand information about colorectal cancer, from understanding the basics to exploring treatment options and what to expect during recovery. We also aim to offer guidance on how to manage the emotional and physical challenges you might face. This book is a resource for you to refer to as you make important decisions, seek support, and work toward recovery.

We'd like to take a moment to acknowledge the many people who made this book possible. To the medical professionals who shared their expertise and insights, thank you for helping us create an informative and accurate resource.

To the colorectal cancer survivors and their families who shared their personal stories, we are grateful for your courage and willingness to inspire others. And to the countless patients and caregivers who have navigated the challenges of colorectal cancer, we are honored to be a part of your journey.

Remember, you are not alone. There are many people and resources available to support you, and we hope this book becomes a trusted companion during this time. As you read through the following chapters, we encourage you to take things one step at a time and to reach out for support whenever you need it.

Thank you for choosing this book, and we wish you strength and hope as you move forward.

About This Guide

This guide is designed to be a comprehensive resource for anyone facing a colorectal cancer diagnosis. It covers a wide range of topics, from understanding what colorectal cancer is to exploring treatment options and learning how to manage the emotional and physical challenges that come with it.

Our aim is to provide you with practical, easy-to-understand information that you can use to make informed decisions about your care and treatment. We understand that being diagnosed with cancer can be overwhelming, and you might have a lot of questions about what comes next. This guide aims to answer those questions and offer helpful tips for navigating each stage of the process.

In this book, you'll find:

- An overview of colorectal cancer, including its causes, symptoms, and diagnostic methods.
- Information on different treatment options and what to expect during each type of treatment.
- Advice on coping with the emotional impact of a cancer diagnosis, as well as guidance for finding support and resources.

- Tips for managing side effects, maintaining a healthy lifestyle, and improving your quality of life during and after treatment.
- Personal stories from cancer survivors to inspire and encourage you.

We understand that each person's experience with colorectal cancer is unique, so we encourage you to use this guide as a flexible resource. Feel free to skip to the sections that are most relevant to you, and refer back to other sections as needed. You might also want to share this guide with family members, friends, or caregivers who are supporting you through your journey.

Remember, this guide is not a substitute for professional medical advice. Always consult your healthcare team for personalized guidance and recommendations. We're here to provide you with information and support, but your doctors and specialists are your best source of advice for your specific situation.

We hope this guide helps you feel more informed, empowered, and supported as you face colorectal cancer. You're not alone in this journey, and we're here to help you every step of the way.

How to Use This Book

This guide is designed to be a comprehensive resource that addresses the many aspects of colorectal cancer. It provides practical information and support to help you navigate this challenging journey. To make the most of this book, here's a guide on how to use it effectively:

1. Start Where You Are Comfortable

This book is structured to allow you to start wherever feels most relevant to you. If you're newly diagnosed and want to understand the basics of colorectal cancer, start with the first few chapters. If you're looking for information on treatment options or coping strategies, you can skip ahead to those sections. There's no right or wrong way to use this book.

2. Use the Table of Contents and Index

The table of contents at the beginning of the book lists all the chapters and their topics. Use it to find the sections that interest you the most. Additionally, there's an index at the back of the book to help you quickly locate specific terms or topics.

This can be useful when you're looking for specific information or need a quick reference.

3. Take Notes and Highlight

As you read through the book, you might find certain information especially useful or relevant to your situation. Feel free to take notes in the margins or use sticky notes to mark important pages. Highlighting key points can also help you quickly revisit information that stood out to you.

4. Share with Family and Caregivers

Dealing with colorectal cancer involves a support network, which might include family, friends, orc caregivers. Consider sharing relevant sections of this book with them so they can better understand what you're going through and how they can help.

5. Remember It's a Guide, Not a Substitute for Medical Advice

While this book provides valuable information, it's important to remember that your healthcare team is your primary source of medical advice and guidance. Use this book to supplement the information you receive from your doctors, but always consult with them before making any major decisions about your treatment or care.

6. Revisit Sections as Needed

Your journey with colorectal cancer may evolve over time, and so might your needs. Revisit sections of this book as you progress through treatment and recovery. You might find new insights or guidance that align with your current situation.

We hope this book becomes a valuable resource for you as you navigate the journey with colorectal cancer. It's designed to offer you support, guidance, and information to help you make informed decisions and feel empowered during this challenging time.

Chapter 1: Understanding Colorectal Cancer

What is Colorectal Cancer?

Colorectal cancer is a type of cancer that starts in the colon or rectum, both of which are parts of the large intestine. The colon is a long, tube-like organ that absorbs water and nutrients from food, while the rectum is the final section where waste is stored before leaving the body. Colorectal cancer can develop in either of these areas.

Cancer begins when cells in the body start to grow uncontrollably, forming a lump or mass called a tumor. These tumors can be benign (non-cancerous) or malignant (cancerous). In colorectal cancer, the malignant tumors can grow into surrounding tissues and spread to other parts of the body, a process known as metastasis.

How Does Colorectal Cancer Develop?

Colorectal cancer often starts as small, non-cancerous growths called polyps, which form on the inner lining of the colon or rectum. While many polyps are harmless, some can eventually become cancerous if not removed. That's why regular screening and early detection are crucial in preventing colorectal cancer or catching it at an early stage when treatment is more effective.

Understanding colorectal cancer is the first step in addressing it. With early detection, treatment, and healthy lifestyle choices, it's possible to manage the disease effectively. Remember, always discuss any concerns or questions with your healthcare provider for personalized guidance and advice.

Causes and Risk Factors

Colorectal cancer occurs when cells in the colon or rectum grow abnormally, forming tumors that can invade nearby tissues or spread to other parts of the body. While the exact cause of colorectal cancer isn't always clear, a combination of genetic, lifestyle, and environmental factors can increase the risk of developing the disease.

Causes of Colorectal Cancer

Colorectal cancer usually starts from benign growths called polyps that develop in the colon or rectum. Over time, these polyps can become cancerous due to changes in their genetic material (DNA). DNA contains the instructions for how cells function, and mutations in certain genes can cause cells to grow uncontrollably, leading to cancer.

These genetic changes can be inherited or acquired:

- **Inherited Genetic Changes:** Some people inherit genetic mutations from their parents that increase the risk of colorectal cancer. Conditions like familial adenomatous polyposis (FAP) and Lynch syndrome (hereditary non-polyposis colorectal cancer) are associated with a high risk of developing colorectal cancer.
- **Acquired Genetic Changes**: These changes occur over time due to factors like aging or exposure to certain substances. They are not inherited but can still lead to cancer.

Risk Factors for Colorectal Cancer

A risk factor is anything that increases the likelihood of developing a disease. *Here are some of the key risk factors for colorectal cancer:*

1. Age

Colorectal cancer is more common in people over 50, though it can occur in younger individuals as well.

2. Family History and Genetics

A family history of colorectal cancer increases your risk, especially if close relatives like parents or siblings have had the disease. Inherited genetic conditions like Lynch syndrome also raise the risk.

3. Personal Medical History

If you've had colorectal polyps, inflammatory bowel disease (like Crohn's disease or ulcerative colitis), or certain types of cancer, you're at a higher risk.

4. Lifestyle Factors

Unhealthy lifestyle choices can increase the risk of colorectal cancer:

- *Diet*: A diet high in red meat and processed foods, with low intake of fruits, vegetables, and whole grains, can raise the risk.

- *Physical Inactivity*: Lack of regular exercise is linked to a higher risk of colorectal cancer.
- *Obesity*: Being overweight or obese is another risk factor.
- *Smoking and Alcohol:* Smoking and excessive alcohol consumption can increase the risk.

5. Other Factors

- *Diabetes*: People with type 2 diabetes have a higher risk of colorectal cancer.
- *Ethnicity*: Certain ethnic groups, such as African Americans, may have a higher risk of colorectal cancer.
- *Exposure to Radiation*: People who have had radiation therapy to the abdomen or pelvis for other cancers may have an increased risk.

It's important to remember that having one or more risk factors doesn't mean you'll definitely develop colorectal cancer. Similarly, some people with no known risk factors may still get the disease. Regular screening and healthy lifestyle choices can help reduce the risk and detect the cancer early when it's most treatable. If you're concerned about your risk, discuss it with your healthcare provider to determine the best course of action.

Types of Colorectal Cancer

Colorectal cancer refers to cancer that starts in the colon or rectum. While most cases of colorectal cancer are of a specific type, there are variations in where and how these cancers originate. *Here's an overview of the main types of colorectal cancer and some of the less common forms.*

1. Adenocarcinoma

Adenocarcinoma is by far the most common type of colorectal cancer, accounting for about 95% of all cases. This type of cancer arises from the glandular cells that line the inside of the colon and rectum. These glandular cells are responsible for producing mucus to help move stool through the digestive tract.

Adenocarcinomas are typically divided into two categories:

- ***Mucinous Adenocarcinoma***: This subtype contains a significant amount of mucus and tends to be more aggressive.
- ***Signet Ring Cell Adenocarcinoma***: This rare subtype is named for its appearance under a microscope, where the cells have a distinctive "signet ring" shape due to the large amount of

mucus. It tends to be more aggressive and challenging to treat.

2. Gastrointestinal Stromal Tumors (GISTs)

Gastrointestinal stromal tumors are a rare type of colorectal cancer that originates from cells in the walls of the digestive tract called interstitial cells of Cajal (ICCs). Although GISTs are more commonly found in the stomach or small intestine, they can also occur in the colon or rectum. These tumors are typically treated with surgery and, in some cases, targeted therapy.

3. Lymphomas

Lymphomas are cancers that start in lymphocytes, a type of white blood cell involved in the immune system. While lymphomas usually develop in lymph nodes or other parts of the lymphatic system, they can also occur in the colon or rectum. These cancers require different treatment approaches, such as chemotherapy or radiation therapy.

4. Carcinoid Tumors

Carcinoid tumors are a type of neuroendocrine tumor that can develop in the colon or rectum. These tumors grow from neurocndocrine cells, which are involved in hormone production. Carcinoid tumors are usually slow-growing but can spread to other parts of the body. Treatment options vary depending on the tumor's size, location, and aggressiveness.

5. Squamous Cell Carcinoma

Squamous cell carcinoma is a rare type of colorectal cancer that arises from squamous cells, which are flat cells found in the outer layers of the skin and certain mucous membranes. While it's more common in other parts of the body, like the skin or esophagus, it can occur in the rectum.

6. Other Rare Types

There are other rare types of colorectal cancer, such as leiomyosarcomas and melanomas, but they are extremely uncommon. These cancers have unique characteristics and typically require specialized treatment approaches.

Understanding the type of colorectal cancer is crucial because it influences the treatment approach and prognosis. If you've been diagnosed with colorectal cancer, your healthcare provider will perform various tests to determine the specific type and recommend the best course of action based on that information.

Always consult your medical team for detailed information and personalized advice.

Signs and Symptoms

Colorectal cancer can manifest with a variety of signs and symptoms, though it's important to remember that not everyone will experience them in the same way. Early-stage colorectal cancer might not show obvious symptoms, making regular screenings crucial for early detection. These are some of the common signs and symptoms to watch out for:

1. Changes in Bowel Habits

If you notice a persistent change in your bowel habits, it could be a sign of colorectal cancer. This could include:

- New or worsening constipation
- Frequent diarrhea
- Changes in stool consistency (such as stools becoming narrower than usual)

2. Blood in the Stool

The presence of blood in your stool can be a warning sign. Blood can appear as:

- Bright red, indicating it may be coming from the rectum or lower colon
- Dark red or black, suggesting it's from a higher location in the colon

3. Unexplained Weight Loss

Losing weight without trying, especially if accompanied by other symptoms, can be a red flag. This weight loss may occur due to the body's response to cancer or changes in metabolism.

4. Abdominal Pain or Discomfort

Some people with colorectal cancer experience abdominal pain, cramping, or discomfort. The pain can vary in intensity and may be constant or come and go.

5. Fatigue or Weakness

Persistent fatigue or feeling unusually weak, even with enough rest, can be a symptom of colorectal cancer. This may be related to blood loss, leading to anemia, or the body's response to cancer.

6. Feeling of Incomplete Bowel Movements

If you have a sensation that you haven't fully emptied your bowels, even after going to the bathroom, it could be related to colorectal cancer.

7. Other Symptoms

Though less common, other signs can include:

- Persistent bloating or gas
- A noticeable lump or mass in the abdomen
- Changes in appetite or unexplained nausea

When to See a Doctor

If you experience any of these symptoms persistently, it's important to consult a healthcare provider. While these symptoms can also be caused by other conditions, it's essential to get a proper diagnosis to determine the underlying cause.

Early detection of colorectal cancer can significantly improve treatment outcomes, so don't hesitate to seek medical advice if you have concerns. Your healthcare provider can perform tests to diagnose the cause of your symptoms and recommend the appropriate treatment.

Diagnostic Tests and Screening

Detecting colorectal cancer early is crucial for effective treatment and improved outcomes. Several tests and screening methods are used to identify colorectal cancer, polyps, or other abnormalities in the colon and rectum. Here's an overview of the most common diagnostic tests and screening methods:

1. Colonoscopy

Colonoscopy is considered the gold standard for colorectal cancer screening. In this procedure, a doctor uses a long, flexible tube with a camera (a colonoscope) to examine the entire length of the colon and rectum. If any polyps or suspicious areas are found, the doctor can remove them or take tissue samples (biopsies) for further analysis.

2. Sigmoidoscopy

Sigmoidoscopy is similar to colonoscopy but only examines the lower part of the colon and rectum (the sigmoid colon). It's a shorter procedure and may be used for screening or to follow up on abnormal results from other tests.

3. Fecal Occult Blood Test (FOBT)

The fecal occult blood test checks for hidden (occult) blood in the stool, which could indicate the presence of polyps or colorectal cancer. There are two main types of FOBT: the guaiac-based test and the immunochemical-based test (FIT). Both require you to provide stool samples at home, which are then sent to a lab for analysis.

4. Stool DNA Test (sDNA)

This test analyzes stool samples for specific DNA changes associated with colorectal cancer. It can detect both cancer and large polyps with a high degree of accuracy. A commonly known sDNA test is Cologuard®, which involves collecting a stool sample at home and sending it to a lab for testing.

5. Virtual Colonoscopy (CT Colonography)

Virtual colonoscopy uses a CT scan to create detailed images of the colon and rectum. This non-invasive procedure can identify polyps and other abnormalities. However, if abnormalities are found, a traditional colonoscopy might be needed to remove them or perform a biopsy.

6. Blood Tests

While not used for primary screening, certain blood tests can help in monitoring colorectal cancer or assessing treatment outcomes. For example, the carcinoembryonic antigen (CEA) test measures a protein that can be elevated in colorectal cancer. However, blood tests are not sufficient to diagnose colorectal cancer on their own.

When to Get Screened

The recommended age for beginning colorectal cancer screening is typically 45 to 50, depending on your risk factors and medical history. However, if you have a family history of colorectal cancer, a genetic predisposition, or other risk factors, you may need to start screening earlier. Talk to your healthcare provider to determine the best screening schedule for you.

Regular screening can help detect colorectal cancer early, even before symptoms appear, allowing for more effective treatment and better outcomes. If you have questions about screening, diagnostic tests, or your risk factors, don't hesitate to ask your healthcare provider for guidance.

Chapter 2: Treatment Options

Overview of Treatment Approaches

The treatment of colorectal cancer varies depending on the stage of the cancer, its location, and other individual factors. Below are the most frequently used treatment methods:

1. Surgery: Surgery is typically the primary treatment for colorectal cancer, especially when it's localized. The aim is to remove the cancer along with a margin of healthy tissue to ensure all cancerous cells are taken out.

Types of surgery include:

- **Polypectomy**: Removing polyps during a colonoscopy or sigmoidoscopy.

- **Local Excision:** Removing small tumors along with surrounding tissue.

- **Colectomy**: Removing part or all of the colon, sometimes with the creation of a colostomy or ileostomy to divert waste.

2. Chemotherapy: Chemotherapy uses drugs to kill or slow the growth of cancer cells. It can be administered before surgery to shrink tumors (neoadjuvant), after surgery to destroy any remaining cancer cells (adjuvant), or to treat advanced or metastatic colorectal cancer to slow disease progression and manage symptoms.

3. Radiation Therapy: Radiation therapy uses high-energy beams to destroy cancer cells. It's often used in rectal cancer, either before surgery to reduce tumor size or after surgery to lower the risk of recurrence. In more severe instances, radiation therapy can be used to ease symptoms.

4. Targeted Therapy: Targeted therapy aims at particular molecules that play a role in the progression of cancer. These drugs aim to affect only the cancer cells, which may lead to fewer side effects compared to traditional chemotherapy. Targeted therapy is typically used for advanced colorectal cancer, especially when specific genetic mutations are present.

5. Immunotherapy: Immunotherapy boosts the immune system to fight cancer. It's generally used for colorectal cancers with specific genetic characteristics, such as high microsatellite instability (MSI-H) or mismatch repair deficiency (dMMR).

6. Clinical Trials: Clinical trials test new treatments or treatment combinations. Participating in a clinical trial may give patients access to emerging therapies that are not yet widely available. Clinical trials can be an option for patients who have not responded to standard treatments.

Choosing the Right Treatment: The choice of treatment depends on the cancer's stage, location, the patient's health, and personal preferences. Often, a combination of treatments is used to achieve the best outcome. Discussing the available options with your healthcare team will help you understand which treatments are most appropriate for you.

Surgery

Surgery is a common treatment for colorectal cancer, especially when the cancer is detected early. The type of surgery and specific procedures used depend on the size, location, and stage of the cancer. Here are the main types of surgeries and their procedures for colorectal cancer:

1. Polypectomy: Polypectomy involves removing small polyps from the lining of the colon or rectum during a colonoscopy or sigmoidoscopy. This procedure is typically used for early-stage colorectal cancer when the cancer is confined to a polyp.

2. Local Excision: Local excision is a surgical procedure where a small area of tissue containing the cancer is removed. It's generally used when the tumor is in the rectum and is small enough to be removed without major surgery.

3. Colectomy: A colectomy involves removing part or all of the colon. There are different types of colectomies:

- **Partial Colectomy**: This procedure removes only the part of the colon containing cancer. It's also known as a segmental resection.

- **Total Colectomy**: This involves removing the entire colon. It's less common and is typically used when there are multiple areas of concern or when cancer has spread extensively.

4. *Proctectomy*: A proctectomy is the surgical removal of the rectum. It's used when the cancer is located in the rectum. Depending on the extent of the removal, a temporary or permanent stoma (an opening in the abdomen for waste to leave the body) may be needed.

5. *Colostomy and Ileostomy*: Sometimes, after a colectomy or proctectomy, a colostomy or ileostomy is required. These procedures create a stoma, allowing waste to be collected in an external pouch:

- **Colostomy**: The stoma is created from the colon.

- **Ileostomy**: The stoma is created from the ileum, the last part of the small intestine.

6. *Laparoscopic and Robotic Surgery*: Laparoscopic surgery uses small incisions and special instruments to perform the procedure, reducing recovery time and post-operative pain. Robotic surgery is a type of laparoscopic surgery where the surgeon controls robotic arms to perform the operation with high precision.

7. Resection with Anastomosis: In this procedure, a portion of the colon or rectum is removed, and the remaining ends are reconnected (anastomosis) to maintain the digestive tract's continuity. This is commonly used in partial colectomies or proctectomies.

8. Choosing the Right Surgery: The choice of surgical procedure depends on the cancer's location, size, and stage, as well as the patient's overall health and personal preferences. Surgeons often consider minimally invasive techniques, like laparoscopic or robotic surgery, to reduce recovery time and complications.

If you're facing surgery for colorectal cancer, your healthcare team will discuss the options with you and help determine the best approach for your situation.

Chemotherapy

Chemotherapy is a treatment that uses powerful drugs to kill cancer cells or stop them from growing and spreading. In colorectal cancer, chemotherapy can play different roles depending on the stage of the cancer, the treatment goals, and individual factors. This is a guide on how chemotherapy is used in colorectal cancer:

1. Adjuvant Chemotherapy: Adjuvant chemotherapy is given after surgery to eliminate any remaining cancer cells and reduce the risk of the cancer returning.

This approach is commonly used when the cancer is more advanced or when there's a risk that cancer cells may have spread to nearby lymph nodes.

2. Neoadjuvant Chemotherapy: Neoadjuvant chemotherapy is given before surgery to shrink the tumor, making it easier to remove. This approach is often used for rectal cancer to reduce the tumor size, which can lead to more successful surgeries and lower rates of recurrence.

3. Palliative Chemotherapy: Palliative chemotherapy is used when the cancer has spread to other parts of the body (metastatic colorectal cancer). While it may not cure the cancer, it aims to control its growth, reduce symptoms, and improve quality of life.

4. Chemotherapy Drugs Several chemotherapy drugs are used to treat colorectal cancer. Common drugs include:

- **Fluorouracil (5-FU):** Often combined with other drugs or used with leucovorin to boost its effectiveness.

- **Capecitabine**: An oral chemotherapy drug that converts to 5-FU in the body.

- **Oxaliplatin**: Commonly used in combination with 5-FU and leucovorin (known as FOLFOX).

- **Irinotecan**: Often used in combination with other chemotherapy drugs (like FOLFIRI).

These drugs can be used individually or in combination to enhance their effectiveness. The specific drug regimen depends on the stage of the cancer and the treatment goals.

5. *Side Effects of Chemotherapy*: Chemotherapy can cause side effects because it affects both cancer cells and healthy cells that divide quickly. Common side effects include:

- Fatigue
- Nausea and vomiting
- Hair loss
- Mouth sores
- Diarrhea or constipation
- Increased risk of infection due to reduced white blood cell counts

However, not everyone experiences these side effects, and there are medications and treatments to manage them. Your healthcare team will monitor your response to chemotherapy and help you manage any side effects.

6. *Duration of Chemotherapy*: The length of chemotherapy treatment varies. It can range from several weeks to several months, depending on the regimen and the purpose of the treatment. Chemotherapy is usually given in cycles, with rest periods in between to allow the body to recover.

7. *Monitoring During Chemotherapy*: While undergoing chemotherapy, patients are closely monitored for side effects and treatment effectiveness. Blood tests and imaging studies are often used to track progress and adjust treatment as needed.

Chemotherapy is an important tool in the treatment of colorectal cancer. If it's part of your treatment plan, your healthcare team will work with you to understand the process and address any concerns you have.

Radiation Therapy

Radiation therapy uses high-energy beams or particles to kill cancer cells or prevent them from growing. It is a common treatment for rectal cancer and is sometimes used for colon cancer. Here's a look at how radiation therapy is used in the treatment of colorectal cancer:

1. When Radiation Therapy Is Used Radiation therapy can be used in several scenarios:

- **Neoadjuvant Radiation**: Before surgery to shrink the tumor, making it easier to remove and potentially reducing the risk of recurrence.

- **Adjuvant Radiation**: After surgery to kill any remaining cancer cells and lower the chance of cancer returning.

- **Palliative Radiation:** To relieve symptoms and improve quality of life in cases where the cancer has spread (metastasized) or cannot be fully removed by surgery.

2. Types of Radiation Therapy: There are two main types of radiation therapy used for colorectal cancer:

- **External Beam Radiation** Therapy (EBRT): This is the most common form of radiation therapy. It uses a machine to direct high-energy beams at the cancer from outside the body. Treatment is usually given in a series of sessions over several weeks.

- **Brachytherapy**: Also known as internal radiation therapy, this involves placing a radioactive source near or inside the tumor. Brachytherapy is less commonly used but may be an option for certain rectal cancers.

3. How Radiation Therapy Is Given: Radiation therapy is usually delivered in a healthcare setting, often in daily sessions from Monday to Friday, with rest on weekends. Each session is brief, lasting about 10-30 minutes. The total duration of treatment depends on the therapy's goal and other factors.

4. Side Effects of Radiation Therapy Radiation therapy can cause side effects, as it affects both cancerous and healthy cells.

Common side effects include:
- Skin irritation or redness at the treatment site

- Fatigue
- Diarrhea or changes in bowel habits
- Abdominal discomfort or cramps
- Urinary issues if the radiation affects nearby organs

These side effects vary depending on the location and intensity of the radiation. Fortunately, most side effects are temporary and can be managed with medical support and self-care.

5. *Preparation and Aftercare:* Before radiation therapy begins, a planning session (called simulation) is conducted to determine the exact location to target. This involves imaging scans to map out the treatment area.

During treatment, the patient must remain as still as possible to ensure accurate targeting of the radiation. After treatment, regular follow-ups are essential to monitor for side effects, check the effectiveness of the therapy, and manage any symptoms.

6. *Benefits of Radiation*: Therapy Radiation therapy can be highly effective in reducing tumor size and killing cancer cells, especially when combined with other treatments like surgery or chemotherapy. It can also help relieve pain and other symptoms in advanced cases.

Your healthcare team will guide you through the process and answer any questions you have about radiation therapy. They will also work with you to manage any side effects and ensure the best possible outcome from your treatment.

Targeted Therapy

Targeted therapy is a form of cancer treatment that uses drugs designed to specifically attack certain molecules involved in the growth and spread of cancer cells. Unlike traditional chemotherapy, which affects both cancerous and healthy rapidly dividing cells, targeted therapy aims to focus on cancer cells, potentially reducing side effects. Here's a clear explanation of how targeted therapy is used in the treatment of colorectal cancer:

1. What Is Targeted Therapy? Targeted therapy involves drugs that "target" specific proteins or genes involved in cancer cell growth. These targets are often unique to cancer cells or are present in much higher levels compared to normal cells. This approach can inhibit cancer progression with less damage to healthy cells.

2. When Is Targeted Therapy Used? Targeted therapy is typically used in advanced or metastatic colorectal cancer, where the cancer has spread beyond the colon or rectum. It is often used in combination with other treatments, like chemotherapy, to enhance effectiveness.

3. Common Targets in Colorectal Cancer: In colorectal cancer, certain genetic changes or protein expressions are commonly targeted by specific drugs. Here are a few key targets:

- **Epidermal Growth Factor Receptor (EGFR):** This protein can promote cancer cell growth when overactive. Drugs that target EGFR, such as cetuximab and panitumumab, can slow the growth of these cancer cells.

- **Vascular Endothelial Growth Factor (VEGF):** This protein helps cancer cells create new blood vessels (angiogenesis), providing nutrients for growth. Drugs that target VEGF, like bevacizumab, aim to restrict this blood vessel formation.

- **BRAF and RAS Mutations**: Some colorectal cancers have mutations in genes like BRAF and RAS. Targeted therapies such as vemurafenib (for BRAF mutations) or specific RAS inhibitors can be used to treat these cancers.

4. Side Effects of Targeted Therapy Targeted therapy is generally more specific than chemotherapy, but it can still cause side effects. Common side effects include:

- Skin rash or irritation
- Fatigue
- Diarrhea
- High blood pressure
- Increased risk of infection

The severity of side effects varies depending on the drug and the individual's response to treatment. Healthcare teams monitor patients closely to manage these effects.

5. Choosing the Right Targeted Therapy: Before starting targeted therapy, genetic testing of the tumor is often performed to identify specific mutations or markers. This helps determine which targeted therapy may be most effective for a particular patient. Not all colorectal cancers respond to targeted therapy, so these tests are critical in guiding treatment decisions.

6. Integration with Other Treatments: Targeted therapy is often used alongside other treatments, like chemotherapy or radiation therapy, to improve outcomes. It can also be part of a treatment plan for patients in clinical trials, where new targeted drugs or combinations are being tested.

If targeted therapy is part of your treatment plan, your healthcare team will explain the specific drugs used, how they work, and what to expect during treatment. They will also monitor your response and adjust the therapy as needed.

Immunotherapy

Immunotherapy is a type of cancer treatment that aims to harness the body's immune system to fight cancer cells. Unlike traditional treatments that directly target cancer cells, immunotherapy stimulates or modifies the immune system to recognize and attack cancer more effectively. In colorectal cancer, immunotherapy can be a valuable option for certain patients. Here's an overview of immunotherapy and its role in treating colorectal cancer:

1. What Is Immunotherapy? Immunotherapy involves various techniques to boost or modulate the immune system's ability to detect and destroy cancer cells. This can include the use of specific drugs, known as immune checkpoint inhibitors, that help the immune system to "see" and respond to cancer cells.

2. When Is Immunotherapy Used? Immunotherapy is often used to treat advanced or metastatic colorectal cancer, especially in cases with specific genetic markers. It can be part of a broader treatment plan or a standalone option depending on the nature of the cancer.

3. Key Types of Immunotherapy: There are several types of immunotherapy used in colorectal cancer. The most common type is immune checkpoint inhibitors, which block proteins that prevent immune cells from attacking cancer cells. The key immune checkpoint inhibitors in colorectal cancer are:

- **PD-1 Inhibitors**: These drugs block the programmed death-1 (PD-1) protein on immune cells, allowing them to attack cancer cells more effectively. Examples include pembrolizumab and nivolumab.

- **CTLA-4 Inhibitors**: This class of drugs targets the cytotoxic T-lymphocyte-associated protein 4 (CTLA-4) to enhance the immune response against cancer cells. Ipilimumab is a commonly used CTLA-4 inhibitor.

4. When Is Immunotherapy Effective? Immunotherapy is most effective in colorectal cancers with specific characteristics, such as:

- **High Microsatellite Instability (MSI-H) or Mismatch Repair Deficiency (dMMR):** These genetic traits indicate a higher likelihood of response to immunotherapy. Patients with these markers are often considered prime candidates for immune checkpoint inhibitors.

5. *Side Effects of Immunotherapy*: While immunotherapy can be effective, it may also cause side effects, often related to the immune system's activation. Common side effects include:

- Fatigue
- Skin rash or itching
- Joint pain or stiffness
- Digestive issues like diarrhea or nausea

In some cases, the immune system may attack healthy organs, leading to more serious side effects. Your healthcare team will monitor you closely for these effects and manage them as needed.

6. Integration with Other Treatments: Immunotherapy can be used alone or in combination with other treatments, such as chemotherapy or targeted therapy, to improve outcomes. It can also be part of clinical trials, where new combinations and applications of immunotherapy are being studied.

If immunotherapy is part of your treatment plan, your healthcare team will guide you through the process and explain what to expect. They will monitor your response to ensure that the treatment is effective and that any side effects are managed promptly.

Clinical Trials and Experimental Treatments

Clinical trials are research studies that test new treatments or new ways of using existing treatments for colorectal cancer. They are crucial for advancing medical knowledge and can offer patients access to innovative therapies that aren't yet widely available. Below are what you need to know about clinical trials and experimental treatments:

1. What Are Clinical Trials? Clinical trials evaluate the safety and effectiveness of new drugs, therapies, or treatment combinations. They follow strict protocols to ensure participant safety and gather reliable data. Clinical trials are typically conducted in several phases, each with a specific goal:

- **Phase I:** Focuses on safety and dosage.
- **Phase II:** Tests effectiveness and further assesses safety.

- **Phase III**: Compares new treatments with standard treatments to establish effectiveness.

- **Phase IV:** Monitors long-term effects and outcomes after a treatment is approved.

2. Why Participate in a Clinical Trial? Patients choose to participate in clinical trials for various reasons:

- **Access to New Treatments**: Clinical trials often provide early access to groundbreaking therapies.

- **Contribution to Medical Research**: Participants help advance scientific understanding of colorectal cancer.

- **Close Medical Monitoring**: Clinical trial participants are closely monitored, ensuring a high level of care and attention.

3. Types of Clinical Trials: Clinical trials for colorectal cancer may test new drugs, targeted therapies, immunotherapy, combination therapies, or novel surgical techniques. Some trials focus on prevention, while others explore better diagnostic methods or new ways to manage side effects.

4. Safety and Informed Consent: Safety is a top priority in clinical trials. Before joining a trial, participants receive detailed information about the treatment, potential risks, benefits, and their rights. This process, called informed consent, ensures patients understand what to expect and agree to participate voluntarily.

5. *How to Find Clinical Trials*: If you're interested in clinical trials, talk to your oncologist or healthcare team. They can guide you to trials that match your specific cancer type, stage, and treatment history. You can also search for clinical trials on websites like ClinicalTrials.gov, which provides a comprehensive list of ongoing trials.

6. *Experimental Treatments*: Experimental treatments are those still in the early stages of research and not yet approved for widespread use. They are usually available only through clinical trials. Examples of experimental treatments for colorectal cancer might include:

- **New targeted therapies**: Drugs designed to target specific genetic mutations or proteins in cancer cells.

- **Advanced immunotherapies**: Innovative ways to boost the immune system's ability to fight cancer.

- **Novel drug combinations**: Exploring new ways to combine existing drugs for enhanced effectiveness.

7. *Things to Consider Before* joining a clinical trial, consider these *factors*:

- **Eligibility**: Each trial has specific criteria that determine who can participate.

- **Location and Time Commitment**: Some trials require frequent visits to a specific location, which can impact your daily life.
- **Costs**: Clinical trials usually cover the treatment costs, but you may need to cover travel and other personal expenses.

If you're considering joining a clinical trial, discuss it with your healthcare team to understand the potential benefits and risks. They can help you determine if a clinical trial is the right option for your colorectal cancer treatment journey.

Chapter 3: Coping with Diagnosis

Emotional Impact of Diagnosis

Receiving a colorectal cancer diagnosis can be overwhelming and bring a range of emotions. It's normal to feel shocked, scared, angry, or even numb. Understanding these emotions and finding healthy ways to cope is an important part of the journey. This is an overview of the emotional impact of a colorectal cancer diagnosis and some tips for managing it:

1. Shock and Disbelief: The initial reaction to a cancer diagnosis is often shock and disbelief. You might feel like you're in a fog or that this can't be happening to you. This is a natural response to unexpected and life-changing news.

2. Fear and Anxiety: Cancer brings uncertainty about the future. You might worry about your health, treatments, and their side effects, or the impact on your family and work. This fear can lead to anxiety, affecting your ability to sleep, eat, or focus on everyday activities.

3. Anger and Frustration: It's common to feel anger or frustration after a diagnosis. You might question why this happened to you, feel anger toward your body for failing you, or frustration with the healthcare system or treatments.

4. Sadness and Grief: A cancer diagnosis can lead to feelings of sadness and grief. You might mourn the loss of your health, worry about missing important life events, or feel sadness for the uncertainty ahead.

5. Loneliness and Isolation: You might feel alone in your diagnosis, as if others can't understand what you're going through. This can lead to isolation, even if you're surrounded by family and friends.

6. Coping with the Emotional Impact: While the emotional impact of a colorectal cancer diagnosis can be intense, there are ways to cope and find support:

- **Talk About Your Feelings:** Sharing your emotions with a trusted friend, family member, or counselor can help you process what you're feeling.

- **Join Support Groups**: Connecting with others who have experienced colorectal cancer can provide a sense of community and understanding.

- **Seek Professional Help:** A therapist or counselor with experience in cancer-related issues can help you navigate complex emotions.

- **Practice Self-Care:** Taking care of your physical and mental health is essential. This can include regular exercise, eating well, getting enough sleep, and practicing relaxation techniques like meditation or deep breathing.

- **Stay Informed:** Knowledge can help reduce anxiety. Ask questions, learn about your condition, and understand your treatment options.

7. Find Meaning and Hope: While a cancer diagnosis can be daunting, many people find strength and meaning in their journey. This might involve setting new goals, rediscovering a sense of purpose, or finding hope in stories of survival and resilience.

Remember, everyone's emotional response to a cancer diagnosis is unique. It's okay to feel a mix of emotions, and there's no right or wrong way to cope. The key is to acknowledge your feelings and seek support when needed. If you or someone you know is struggling with the emotional impact of a colorectal cancer diagnosis, don't hesitate to reach out to a healthcare professional or support organization for guidance and help.

Communicating with Loved Ones

Communicating with family and friends about a colorectal cancer diagnosis can be challenging. It's natural to feel uncertain about how to share such significant news, what to say, and how your loved ones might react. Here are some tips for effectively communicating with those closest to you:

1. Decide Who to Tell and When: Consider who needs to know about your diagnosis and when you'd like to share the news. You might want to start with close family members or friends who can offer support and help you process your emotions. As you feel ready, you can expand the circle to include other loved ones and acquaintances.

2. Choose a Comfortable Setting: Select a setting where you feel at ease and have privacy for your conversations. This might be at home, in a quiet park, or at a close friend's place. A comfortable environment can make the discussion easier for both you and your loved ones.

3. Be Honest and Direct: It's best to be clear and straightforward when sharing your diagnosis. You don't need to go into extensive medical details, but explaining the basics can help your loved ones understand the situation. For example, you might say, "I have been diagnosed with colorectal cancer, and I will need to undergo treatment."

4. Express Your Feelings: Share your emotions openly. Whether you're feeling scared, anxious, or hopeful, expressing your feelings can foster a deeper connection with your loved ones. It's okay to be vulnerable and let others know how they can support you.

5. Encourage Questions: Your loved ones may have questions about your diagnosis, treatment, and what to expect. Encourage them to ask questions and be prepared to answer to the best of your ability. If you don't know the answer, it's okay to say, "I'm not sure, but I can find out."

6. Discuss Support Needs: Let your loved ones know how they can support you during this time. Whether it's accompanying you to appointments, helping with household tasks, or simply being there to listen, clearly communicating your needs can strengthen your support network.

7. Be Prepared for Reactions: People may react differently to the news of your diagnosis. Some may be supportive and empathetic, while others might feel overwhelmed or struggle with their emotions. Give them time to process the information, and don't be afraid to revisit the conversation later if needed.

Finding Support

Support Groups, Counseling, and Online Communities

A colorectal cancer diagnosis can be overwhelming, and finding support can make a significant difference in your journey. Support groups, counseling, and online communities offer various ways to connect with others, share experiences, and gain emotional support. Here's a guide to finding support during your colorectal cancer journey:

1. Support Groups: Support groups bring together people with similar experiences to share stories, advice, and encouragement. Joining a colorectal cancer support group can provide a sense of community and reduce feelings of isolation. Here's what to consider when seeking a support group:

- **In-Person Groups:** Many hospitals, cancer centers, and community organizations host support groups where you can meet others face-to-face.

- **Online Groups**: If attending in person is challenging, online support groups offer a convenient way to connect with others from the comfort of your home.

- **Focus and Structure:** Some groups focus on general cancer support, while others are specific to colorectal cancer or even subtypes like rectal cancer. Choose a group that aligns with your needs.

2. Counseling and Therapy: Counseling and therapy provide professional guidance to help you navigate the emotional challenges of a cancer diagnosis. A licensed therapist or counselor with experience in cancer care can offer personalized support. Here's how counseling can benefit you:

- **Emotional Support:** Counseling can help you process complex emotions, such as fear, anger, and grief, in a safe environment.

- **Coping Strategies**: A counselor can teach you techniques to manage stress, anxiety, and other emotional challenges.

- **Family Counseling**: Some therapists offer sessions for families, helping loved ones understand and support you better.

3. Online Communities: Online communities allow you to connect with a broader network of people experiencing colorectal cancer. These platforms offer flexibility and access to a wealth of shared experiences. Here are some popular features of online communities:

- **Forums and Discussion Boards:** You can ask questions, share your story, and seek advice from others with similar experiences.

- **Social Media Groups:** Platforms like Facebook and Reddit have groups dedicated to colorectal cancer support, where you can engage with a larger audience.

- **Webinars and Virtual Events:** Many organizations host online events, offering educational content and opportunities to connect with experts and peers.

4. Finding the Right Support: Finding the right support depends on your preferences and comfort level. Consider these factors when exploring support options:

- **Confidentiality**: Choose groups and counselors that respect your privacy and confidentiality.

- **Flexibility**: Find a format that fits your schedule, whether it's in-person, virtual, or a mix.

- **Quality and Reputation**: Seek reputable groups and licensed professionals to ensure you receive reliable support.

5. Benefits of Support Groups: Being part of a support group, receiving counseling, or joining an online community can offer several benefits, including:

- **Emotional Comfort**: Knowing you're not alone can reduce feelings of isolation and provide emotional relief.

- **Practical Advice**: Support groups and online communities are great sources of practical tips for managing treatment and side effects.

- **Empowerment**: Sharing experiences and learning from others can empower you to take an active role in your care and treatment decisions.

If you're looking for support, start by asking your healthcare team for recommendations. They often have connections with local support groups, counselors, and online resources. Remember, seeking support is a sign of strength, and finding the right network can make your colorectal cancer journey more manageable.

Managing Fear and Anxiety

A colorectal cancer diagnosis can trigger a wave of fear and anxiety. It's natural to worry about your health, treatment, and the impact on your life and loved ones. Managing these feelings is essential for your well-being as you navigate through treatment and beyond. Here's how you can manage fear and anxiety during your colorectal cancer journey:

1. Acknowledge Your Feelings: It's normal to feel afraid and anxious after a cancer diagnosis. Recognize and accept these feelings without judgment. Trying to suppress or deny them can often make them more intense. Instead, give yourself permission to feel what you're feeling.

2. Learn About Your Condition: Knowledge can help reduce anxiety. Learn about colorectal cancer, your treatment options, and what to expect. However, be cautious about information overload. Rely on reputable sources and ask your healthcare team any questions you have.

3. Establish a Support System: Having a strong support system can significantly reduce fear and anxiety. Reach out to family, friends, and support groups. Share your feelings with people you trust, and let them know how they can support you. If you're comfortable, join a support group for colorectal cancer patients to connect with others who understand what you're going through.

4. Practice Relaxation Techniques: Relaxation techniques can help calm your mind and body, reducing stress and anxiety. Consider trying one or more of the following:

- **Deep Breathing:** Slow, deep breaths can help reduce anxiety and promote relaxation.

- **Meditation and Mindfulness**: These practices can help you focus on the present moment and reduce worry about the future.

- **Yoga or Stretching:** Gentle movement can relieve tension and improve your sense of well-being.

5. Stay Active and Maintain Routine: Physical activity can be a great way to manage anxiety. If you're able, try to include regular exercise in your routine, like walking, swimming, or yoga. Staying active can boost your mood and energy levels. Additionally, maintaining a routine, even a simple one, can provide structure and reduce feelings of uncertainty.

6. Limit Negative Influences: Be mindful of the information you consume and the people you interact with. Avoid negative influences that can increase fear and anxiety, such as excessive news consumption or spending time with people who are unsupportive. Instead, focus on positive, supportive, and uplifting sources of information.

7. Seek Professional Help: If fear and anxiety are affecting your daily life, consider seeking help from a mental health professional. A counselor, therapist, or psychologist with experience in cancer-related issues can offer personalized support and coping strategies. They can also help you address deeper emotional concerns that may arise during your cancer journey.

8. Take It One Step at a Time: The journey through colorectal cancer can be overwhelming, especially if you try to anticipate every step ahead of time. Focus on one day at a time, and set small, achievable goals. Celebrate each accomplishment, no matter how small.

Managing fear and anxiety is an ongoing process. Be patient with yourself, and remember that it's okay to ask for help when you need it. With the right support and coping strategies, you can navigate the emotional challenges of colorectal cancer and find a sense of calm and strength along the way.

Making Treatment Decisions

Deciding on the best course of treatment for colorectal cancer is a crucial step in your journey. With various options available, it can be challenging to determine which treatment is best for you. The process involves weighing the benefits and risks, considering personal preferences, and working closely with your healthcare team. Here's a guide to help you navigate the decision-making process for colorectal cancer treatment:

1. Understand Your Diagnosis: Start by understanding the specifics of your diagnosis. Key factors that influence treatment decisions include:

- **Stage of Cancer:** Determines how advanced the cancer is and whether it has spread.

- **Location**: Whether the cancer is in the colon, rectum, or both.

- **Genetic and Molecular Markers:** Certain genetic traits can impact treatment options and outcomes.

Your oncologist can help explain your diagnosis and what it means for your treatment plan.

2. Learn About Treatment Options: Colorectal cancer treatment can involve surgery, chemotherapy, radiation therapy, targeted therapy, immunotherapy, or a combination of these. Learn about each option to understand how they work, their potential side effects, and their success rates. Consider asking your doctor questions like:

- What treatments are available for my specific diagnosis?

- What are the risks and benefits of each treatment?

- What side effects can I expect?

3. Consider Your Goals and Preferences: Your treatment decisions should align with your personal goals and values. Consider factors like:

- **Quality of Life:** How will the treatment affect your day-to-day life, work, and relationships?

- **Length of Treatment:** How long is the treatment process, and what is the expected timeline?

- **Your Health and Fitness**: Are there health conditions or factors that might influence treatment choices?

4. Involve Your Healthcare Team: Your healthcare team, including your oncologist, surgeon, and radiation oncologist, plays a central role in guiding your treatment decisions. Trust their expertise, and don't hesitate to ask questions or seek clarification. If you're unsure about the recommended treatment, consider getting a second opinion to gain additional perspectives.

5. Consider Clinical Trials: Clinical trials can offer access to new and innovative treatments. Ask your doctor if there are clinical trials available that are suitable for your specific cancer type and stage. Participating in a clinical trial may be an option if you're interested in exploring experimental treatments.

6. Weigh the Risks and Benefits: Every treatment comes with potential risks and benefits. Work with your healthcare team to understand these and assess which treatment option aligns best with your goals. This includes considering short-term and long-term side effects, recovery time, and the potential for cancer recurrence.

7. Seek Support and Guidance: Making treatment decisions can be stressful, and you don't have to do it alone. Share your thoughts and concerns with family, friends, or support groups. Talking with others who have experienced colorectal cancer can provide valuable insights and support.

8. Take Your Time: While some treatment decisions need to be made quickly, it's okay to take the time you need to feel comfortable with your choices. Don't rush the process, and remember that you can always revisit your decision if circumstances change.

Ultimately, the goal is to choose a treatment plan that offers the best chance of success while aligning with your values and preferences. With the support of your healthcare team and loved ones, you can make informed treatment decisions that give you the best opportunity for a successful outcome.

Chapter 4: Navigating Treatment

Preparing for Treatment

Preparing for colorectal cancer treatment involves more than just getting medical tests and following your doctor's instructions. It also means preparing yourself emotionally, organizing your daily life, and ensuring you have the support you need. This is a guide to help you get ready for your treatment journey:

1. Understand Your Treatment Plan: Your treatment plan may involve surgery, chemotherapy, radiation therapy, targeted therapy, immunotherapy, or a combination of these. Start by understanding the details of your plan, including:

- What type of treatment you'll receive

- How often you'll need treatment

- Where the treatment will take place

- How long the treatment course will be

Ask your healthcare team to explain the process, expected side effects, and what you need to do to prepare for each treatment session.

2. *Organize Your Medical Information*: Keep all your medical information organized and accessible. This can include:

- Your diagnosis details

- Treatment plan and schedule

- Contact information for your healthcare team

- A list of medications you're taking

Having this information handy can help you stay on track and make it easier to communicate with your healthcare providers.

3. *Arrange for Support:* Having a strong support system is crucial during treatment. Consider:

- **Family and Friends:** Let them know about your treatment schedule and how they can help. This might include providing transportation, preparing meals, or just being there to talk.

- **Support Groups**: Joining a colorectal cancer support group can connect you with others who are going through similar experiences.

- **Professional Help:** Consider enlisting the help of a counselor or therapist to manage stress and anxiety during treatment.

4. *Plan for Time Off Work:* If you're employed, you may need to take time off work for treatment and recovery. Talk to your employer about your situation and understand your rights regarding medical leave. If needed, work with your healthcare team to obtain the necessary medical documentation.

5. *Prepare Your Home:* Make your home as comfortable as possible for your treatment and recovery. Knowing what to expect can help you prepare and reduce anxiety.

- **Comfortable Space:** Create a space where you can rest and relax after treatment sessions.
- **Transportation**: Arrange for reliable transportation to and from treatment appointments.
- **Supplies:** Stock up on essentials like groceries, medications, and other items you'll need during treatment.

6. *Focus on Nutrition and Health:* A healthy diet can help you maintain your strength and energy during treatment. Consult with a dietitian or nutritionist for guidance on foods that are good for your health. Staying hydrated and eating balanced meals can support your immune system and help you recover from treatment.

7. Take Care of Yourself Emotionally: Preparing for treatment can be emotionally challenging. Find healthy ways to cope with stress and anxiety, such as:

- **Relaxation Techniques**: Practice deep breathing, meditation, or gentle yoga to reduce stress.

- **Hobbies and Activities**: Engage in activities that bring you joy and relaxation.

- **Open Communication**: Talk about your feelings with your loved ones, support groups, or a counselor.

8. Understand Financial and Insurance Considerations: Cancer treatment can be costly, so ensure you understand your insurance coverage and any out-of-pocket expenses you may incur. If you need financial assistance, inquire about programs that can help with medical costs, transportation, or other needs.

By taking the time to prepare for treatment, you'll set yourself up for a smoother experience and be better equipped to manage any challenges that come your way. With the right planning, support, and self-care, you'll be ready to face your colorectal cancer treatment with confidence.

Managing Side Effects

Side effects are a common part of colorectal cancer treatment, whether you're undergoing surgery, chemotherapy, radiation therapy, or other therapies. They can vary in type and severity, but there are strategies to help you manage them effectively. Here's a guide to understanding and handling side effects during treatment:

1. Understand Your Side Effects: Different treatments can cause different side effects. Being aware of what to anticipate can assist you in getting ready and lowering anxiety. Common side effects include:

- **Fatigue:** Feeling tired or lacking energy, which can affect daily activities.

- **Nausea and Vomiting**: Often associated with chemotherapy.

- **Diarrhea or Constipation**: Can occur due to medication or changes in diet.

- **Hair Loss:** Typically related to chemotherapy.

- **Mouth Sores:** Ulcers or sores in the mouth, making eating and speaking difficult.

- Skin Changes: Radiation therapy can cause skin irritation, while chemotherapy may cause sensitivity or rashes.

Your healthcare team can provide more information about which side effects you might experience based on your treatment plan.

2. Communicate with Your Healthcare Team: Keep your healthcare team informed about any side effects you experience. They can offer advice, prescribe medications, or adjust your treatment to help manage them. Don't hesitate to report new or worsening symptoms.

3. Manage Fatigue: Fatigue is common, especially during chemotherapy and radiation therapy. To manage fatigue:

- **Rest**: Allow yourself time to rest and recover between activities.

- **Exercise**: Light exercise, like walking or stretching, can boost energy levels.

- **Prioritize Activities**: Focus on the most important tasks and delegate others.

4. Control Nausea and Vomiting: Nausea can be a significant side effect of chemotherapy. To control it:

- **Medications**: Your doctor can prescribe anti-nausea medications to take before or after treatment.

- **Diet**: Eat smaller meals, avoid spicy or greasy foods, and choose bland foods like crackers or toast.

- **Hydration**: Stay hydrated to prevent dehydration caused by vomiting.

5. Handle Diarrhea and Constipation: These digestive issues are common during treatment. To manage them:

- **Diarrhea**: Avoid dairy, caffeine, and high-fiber foods. Use anti-diarrheal medications if prescribed.

- **Constipation**: Increase fiber intake, drink plenty of water, and consider stool softeners or laxatives as directed by your doctor.

6. Care for Your Skin and Hair: Radiation therapy and chemotherapy can affect your skin and hair. To manage these changes:

- **Skin Care:** Use gentle, fragrance-free moisturizers and avoid sun exposure. Wear loose clothing to prevent irritation.

- **Hair Care**: If you're experiencing hair loss, consider wearing hats or wigs. Use mild shampoos and avoid heat styling.

7. Address Mouth Sores: Mouth sores can make eating and speaking difficult. To manage them:

- **Oral Hygiene**: Brush gently with a soft toothbrush and use alcohol-free mouthwash.

- **Diet**: Avoid spicy, acidic, or hot foods. Choose soft, cool foods like yogurt and smoothies.

- **Medications**: Your doctor may prescribe pain-relief gels or mouthwashes to ease discomfort.

8. Seek Emotional Support: Dealing with side effects can be emotionally challenging. Find support through:

- **Counseling**: A therapist or counselor can help you cope with the emotional impact of side effects.

- **Support Groups:** Connect with others who understand what you're going through.

Managing side effects is an important part of your colorectal cancer treatment journey. By staying in communication with your healthcare team, practicing self-care, and seeking support when needed, you can navigate the challenges and focus on your recovery and well-being.

Nutrition and Diet During Treatment

Eating a balanced diet is essential for maintaining your strength and energy during colorectal cancer treatment. Proper nutrition can help you manage side effects, support your immune system, and improve your recovery. Things you need to know about nutrition and diet during colorectal cancer treatment:

1. Importance of Good Nutrition: Nutrition plays a key role in helping your body withstand the effects of treatment. It can:

- Provide energy to maintain daily activities
- Support tissue healing and recovery
- Boost the immune system to fight infections
- Help manage treatment side effects

2. Key Components of a Healthy Diet: During treatment, aim for a well-balanced diet that includes:

- **Proteins**: Found in lean meats, poultry, fish, eggs, beans, and dairy. Proteins are vital for tissue repair and maintaining muscle mass.

- **Carbohydrates**: Sources like whole grains, fruits, and vegetables provide energy.

- **Healthy Fats:** Include sources like avocados, nuts, seeds, and olive oil for additional energy and heart health.

- **Vitamins and Minerals**: Fruits and vegetables are rich in these nutrients, which support overall health.

- **Hydration**: Drink plenty of water, herbal teas, and other non-caffeinated beverages to stay hydrated.

3. *Adjusting Your Diet for Side Effects:* Colorectal cancer treatment can cause various side effects that affect eating and digestion. Here's how to adjust your diet to manage them:

- **Nausea and Vomiting**: Eat small, frequent meals. Choose bland foods like crackers, toast, and applesauce. Ginger tea or ginger chews can help reduce nausea.

- **Diarrhea**: Avoid high-fiber foods and dairy products. Focus on binding foods like bananas, rice, apples, and toast. Stay hydrated with clear fluids.

- **Constipation**: Boost your fiber consumption by incorporating whole grains, fruits, and vegetables into your diet. Drink plenty of water and stay active to help promote regularity.

- **Mouth Sores:** Choose soft foods that are easy to chew and swallow. Avoid spicy, acidic, or hot foods that could irritate the sores.

- **Loss of Appetite**: Eat smaller portions more frequently. Try high-calorie snacks and drinks like smoothies or milkshakes to increase caloric intake.

4. Seeking Professional Guidance: A registered dietitian or nutritionist can be an invaluable resource during treatment.

They can help you create a personalized nutrition plan based on your needs, preferences, and treatment side effects. Ask your healthcare team to refer you to a nutrition specialist if needed.

5. *Safety and Food Hygiene:* During treatment, your immune system may be weakened, so it's crucial to follow food safety guidelines. Here's how to ensure food is safe:

- **Wash Hands and Produce**: Always wash your hands before handling food, and wash fruits and vegetables thoroughly.

- **Cook Food Thoroughly**: Ensure meats, poultry, and fish are cooked to the appropriate temperatures to avoid foodborne illness.

- **Avoid Raw or Undercooked Foods**: Stay away from raw eggs, sushi, or rare meats, as they can increase the risk of infection.

6. *Listen to Your Body*: Every person responds differently to treatment, so it's essential to listen to your body and adjust your diet accordingly. If a particular food or drink makes you feel unwell, avoid it and try alternatives. Be flexible and focus on what makes you feel comfortable and nourished.

Good nutrition can make a significant difference during colorectal cancer treatment. By eating a balanced diet, managing side effects, and seeking professional guidance when needed, you can support your body through treatment and improve your overall well-being.

Exercise and Physical Activity

Regular exercise and physical activity can play a beneficial role during and after colorectal cancer treatment. It helps maintain muscle strength, manage side effects, and improve overall well-being. Here's how you can incorporate exercise into your routine, even during treatment:

1. Benefits of Exercise: Exercise offers many benefits for those undergoing colorectal cancer treatment, including:

- **Improved Energy**: Physical activity can boost your energy levels and reduce fatigue.

- **Reduced Stress and Anxiety**: Exercise can help manage stress and promote a positive mood.

- **Better Sleep**: Regular activity can lead to improved sleep quality.

- **Enhanced Recovery**: Exercise can support muscle strength and flexibility, aiding in recovery after treatment.

- **Reduced Treatment Side Effects:** Regular activity may help manage side effects like nausea and constipation.

2. Types of Exercise: Choose activities that are enjoyable and appropriate for your current fitness level. Consider these types of exercise:

- **Aerobic Exercise:** Activities like walking, swimming, cycling, or light jogging can improve cardiovascular health.

- **Strength Training:** Light weights or resistance bands help maintain muscle mass and strength.

- **Flexibility and Balance**: Stretching, yoga, or tai chi can improve flexibility, balance, and reduce stress.

3. Starting Slowly and Gradually Increasing: If you're new to exercise or have taken a break, start slowly and increase your activity level gradually. Begin with low-impact activities, such as walking or gentle stretching, and build up to more intense exercises as you gain strength and confidence.

4. Listen to Your Body: It's important to listen to your body and not overexert yourself. Pay attention to signs of fatigue or discomfort, and adjust your activity accordingly. If you feel unwell or experience pain, stop exercising and rest. Talk to your healthcare team if you're unsure about the intensity or type of exercise that's safe for you.

5. Make Exercise Part of Your Routine: Consistency is key to gaining the benefits of exercise. Find ways to incorporate physical activity into your daily routine. This could be as simple as taking a walk after dinner or doing light stretches in the morning. Choose activities you enjoy to make exercise feel less like a chore.

6. Get Approval from Your Healthcare Team: Before starting or resuming exercise, get approval from your healthcare team. They can advise on suitable activities based on your treatment plan and overall health. They can also guide you on any precautions to take to ensure your safety.

7. Exercise with Others: Exercising with a friend, family member, or in a group can make physical activity more enjoyable. It also provides an opportunity to socialize and stay motivated. Consider joining a fitness class designed for cancer patients, or ask a friend to join you for a walk or workout session.

8. Set Realistic Goals: Set achievable goals for your exercise routine. This might include exercising a certain number of days per week or walking a specific distance. Celebrate your accomplishments, no matter how small, and adjust your goals as you progress.

Regular exercise can have a positive impact on your colorectal cancer treatment journey. It can improve your energy, mood, and overall quality of life. By choosing activities you enjoy, starting slowly, and getting guidance from your healthcare team, you can create an exercise routine that supports your well-being during and after treatment.

Integrative Therapies and Complementary Medicine

Integrative therapies and complementary medicine are approaches that can be used alongside traditional cancer treatments to improve quality of life and help manage symptoms. They focus on the whole person—mind, body, and spirit—and aim to support the body's healing process. Here's an overview of integrative therapies and complementary medicine for colorectal cancer, including their benefits and common types.

1. What Are Integrative Therapies? Integrative therapies combine conventional medical treatments with complementary practices to address a wide range of needs. The goal is to enhance overall well-being and improve the patient's experience during cancer treatment. Unlike alternative medicine, which is used in place of conventional treatment, integrative therapies are used alongside it.

2. Benefits of Integrative Therapies: Integrative therapies can offer several benefits to colorectal cancer patients:

- **Symptom Management:** They can help manage side effects like pain, nausea, fatigue, and stress.

- **Improved Quality of Life:** Integrative therapies focus on enhancing comfort, relaxation, and emotional well-being.

- **Complement to Conventional Treatments:** These therapies can support recovery and improve the effectiveness of traditional treatments.

3. *Common Integrative Therapies and Complementary Medicine*: Here are some popular integrative therapies that colorectal cancer patients might find beneficial:

- **Acupuncture:** This ancient practice uses thin needles inserted into specific points on the body to relieve pain, reduce nausea, and improve overall energy flow. It can be helpful for managing chemotherapy-induced nausea and neuropathy.

- **Massage Therapy:** Massage can enhance relaxation, alleviate muscle tension, and boost circulation. It may help alleviate stress and anxiety while offering physical comfort.

- **Meditation and Mindfulness:** Techniques such as meditation and mindfulness can aid in reducing stress and enhancing focus. They can also support emotional well-being during challenging times.

- **Yoga and Tai Chi:** These gentle forms of exercise combine physical movement with mindfulness and deep breathing. They can enhance flexibility, balance, and mental clarity.

- **Aromatherapy**: Using essential oils for relaxation and stress relief, aromatherapy can help create a calming environment during treatment and recovery.

- **Nutritional Counseling:** A registered dietitian with experience in cancer care can offer dietary advice to support health and manage treatment-related side effects.

- **Music and Art Therapy**: Creative therapies like music and art can be therapeutic, providing an outlet for expression and reducing stress.

4. Safety and Communication: While integrative therapies can be beneficial, it's crucial to use them safely and in conjunction with conventional treatment.

Here's what to keep in mind:

- **Consult Your Healthcare Team:** Before trying any integrative therapy, discuss it with your oncologist or healthcare provider to ensure it doesn't interfere with your treatment.

- **Use Qualified Practitioners:** Choose licensed or certified practitioners who have experience working with cancer patients.

- **Monitor Your Response**: Pay attention to how your body responds to these therapies and report any adverse effects to your healthcare team.

Integrative therapies and complementary medicine can be valuable tools for enhancing well-being during colorectal cancer treatment. By choosing safe, evidence-based approaches and working closely with your healthcare team, you can enjoy the benefits of these therapies without compromising your primary treatment plan.

Chapter 5: Recovery and Rehabilitation

Post-Treatment Care

Completing treatment for colorectal cancer is a significant milestone, but it's not the end of your journey. Post-treatment care focuses on recovery, monitoring for recurrence, and improving your quality of life. Here are some essential aspects of post-treatment care for colorectal cancer survivors.

1. Follow-Up Appointments: After treatment, you'll need regular follow-up appointments with your healthcare team. These visits monitor your recovery, check for signs of recurrence, and manage any lingering side effects. During these appointments, you might have physical exams, blood tests, or imaging scans. Make sure to keep these appointments and report any new or unusual symptoms to your doctor.

2. Manage Side Effects: Even after treatment, you may experience side effects like fatigue, digestive issues, or nerve damage. Talk to your healthcare team about any ongoing side effects. They can recommend medications, physical therapy, or other interventions to help you manage them. Don't hesitate to ask for help if side effects are affecting your quality of life.

3. Maintain a Healthy Lifestyle: Embracing a healthy lifestyle can aid in your recovery and lower the chance of recurrence. Concentrate on consuming a balanced diet that includes plenty of fruits, vegetables, and whole grains. Maintain physical activity with exercises such as walking, swimming, or yoga, aiming for at least 30 minutes of moderate exercise most days. Additionally, reduce alcohol intake and refrain from smoking.

4. Monitor for Recurrence: One of the primary goals of post-treatment care is to monitor for cancer recurrence. Know the signs and symptoms that might indicate a recurrence, such as unexplained weight loss, abdominal pain, or changes in bowel habits. If you observe any of these symptoms, reach out to your healthcare provider right away. Early detection can significantly impact outcomes if the cancer returns.

5. Address Emotional and Mental Health: Cancer treatment can take a toll on your emotional and mental health. Seek support from counselors, support groups, or mental health professionals if you're experiencing anxiety, depression, or stress. Connecting with other cancer survivors can also be helpful, as they understand the unique challenges of post-treatment life.

6. Rebuild Your Strength and Energy: Recovery after colorectal cancer treatment may take time. Focus on rebuilding your strength and energy at your own pace. Start with light activities and gradually increase your stamina. Give yourself time to rest and recover as necessary. Keep in mind that healing is a process, and it's perfectly fine to progress gradually, one step at a time.

7. Stay Informed and Involved: Stay informed about your condition and follow your healthcare team's advice for post-treatment care. If you have questions or concerns, don't hesitate to ask. Being actively involved in your care can help you feel more in control and confident as you navigate life after treatment.

8. Return to Work and Social Activities: Returning to work and social activities can be a significant step in your post-treatment journey. Talk to your employer about any accommodations you might need, such as flexible hours or a gradual return to work. Reconnecting with friends and engaging in hobbies can help you regain a sense of normalcy and improve your overall well-being.

9. Celebrate Your Achievements: Completing cancer treatment is a huge accomplishment. Take time to celebrate your achievements, whether it's finishing a round of chemotherapy, recovering from surgery, or simply feeling better. Each milestone is a testament to your strength and resilience.

Post-treatment care is about finding a new normal and embracing life after colorectal cancer. By staying connected with your healthcare team, maintaining a healthy lifestyle, and addressing your emotional needs, you can focus on your recovery and enjoy a fulfilling life.

Monitoring for Recurrence

After completing treatment for colorectal cancer, the risk of recurrence can be a significant concern. Monitoring for recurrence involves regular check-ups and tests to detect any signs of cancer returning, which allows for early intervention and improved outcomes. Here's what you need to know about monitoring for recurrence after colorectal cancer treatment.

1. Follow-Up Appointments: Your healthcare team will schedule regular follow-up appointments to monitor your health and check for signs of recurrence. The frequency of these visits depends on factors such as the stage of your cancer, the type of treatment you received, and your overall health. Typically, you'll have follow-up appointments every three to six months for the first few years, then less frequently as time goes on.

2. Blood Tests: Blood tests can be a useful tool in monitoring for recurrence. One common test measures the levels of carcinoembryonic antigen (CEA), a protein that can be elevated in people with colorectal cancer. An increase in CEA levels might indicate a recurrence, but it's not always conclusive. Your doctor may also check other blood markers to assess your health.

3. Imaging Scans: Imaging scans are often used to detect cancer recurrence. These may include:

- **CT Scans:** Provide detailed images of the inside of your body to check for abnormal growths.

- **MRI Scans**: Use magnetic fields to create detailed images, often used to examine the liver and other organs for metastases.

- **PET Scans:** Can detect areas of increased metabolic activity, which might indicate cancer cells.

Your healthcare team will determine which scans are appropriate based on your specific case and follow a regular schedule for these tests.

4. *Colonoscopy:* A colonoscopy is a key tool in monitoring for recurrence, particularly if you had polyps removed during your initial treatment. It allows your doctor to examine the inside of your colon and rectum for any signs of new growths or abnormalities. The timing of colonoscopies depends on your risk factors and the results of previous examinations.

5. *Recognize Signs and Symptoms of Recurrence*: It's important to be aware of potential signs and symptoms of colorectal cancer recurrence. These can include:

- Changes in bowel habits (such as constipation or diarrhea)
- Blood in the stool
- Abdominal pain or discomfort
- Unexplained weight loss
- Fatigue

If you experience any of these symptoms, contact your healthcare provider immediately. Early detection of recurrence can lead to more effective treatment options.

6. *Communicate with Your Healthcare Team*: Maintaining open communication with your healthcare team is crucial in monitoring for recurrence. Share any concerns or symptoms with your doctor, and don't hesitate to ask questions about your follow-up care plan. Your team can help you understand what to expect during each stage of monitoring and what tests are necessary.

7. *Manage Stress and Anxiety*: The fear of recurrence can cause significant stress and anxiety. Find healthy ways to manage these feelings, such as talking to a counselor, joining a support group, or practicing relaxation techniques like meditation or deep breathing. Your healthcare team can also recommend resources to help you cope with the emotional challenges of monitoring for recurrence.

Monitoring for recurrence is an essential part of life after colorectal cancer treatment. By attending regular follow-up appointments, undergoing necessary tests, and staying in communication with your healthcare team, you can increase the chances of early detection and take proactive steps toward maintaining your health.

Rehabilitation and Physical Therapy

Rehabilitation and physical therapy are vital components of recovery after colorectal cancer treatment. They help you regain strength, improve mobility, manage side effects, and enhance overall quality of life. Whether you're recovering from surgery, chemotherapy, or radiation therapy, these services can support you in regaining independence and resuming daily activities.

1. The Role of Rehabilitation and Physical: Therapy Rehabilitation involves a range of therapies designed to restore function and mobility. Physical therapy is a key part of rehabilitation, focusing on exercises and techniques to strengthen muscles, improve flexibility, and increase endurance. It can also help with pain management and reduce the risk of injury.

2. When to Start Rehabilitation: The timing of rehabilitation depends on your treatment and recovery plan. In some cases, rehabilitation starts during treatment, with light exercises to maintain mobility. After surgery, physical therapy might begin once you're stable and cleared for activity. Consult your healthcare team to determine the best time to start rehabilitation.

3. Benefits of Physical Therapy: Physical therapy offers several benefits for colorectal cancer survivors:

- **Improved Mobility**: Exercises designed to increase range of motion can help you move more freely and with less pain.

- **Enhanced Strength:** Strength-building exercises can help you regain muscle mass and stability.

- **Pain Management**: Techniques such as massage, stretching, and heat therapy can reduce pain and discomfort.

- **Reduced Fatigue:** Regular physical activity can boost energy levels and reduce cancer-related fatigue.

- **Increased Confidence:** As you regain strength and mobility, you'll likely feel more confident in your ability to perform daily activities.

4. Common Physical Therapy Exercises: Physical therapy exercises vary based on individual needs and limitations. Some common exercises for colorectal cancer survivors include:

- **Walking and Light Aerobics**: Helps improve cardiovascular health and endurance.

- **Strength Training:** Focuses on building muscle strength with resistance bands or light weights.

- **Balance and Coordination Exercises**: Aims to improve stability and reduce the risk of falls.

- **Stretching and Flexibility Exercises**: Increases flexibility and reduces muscle stiffness.

5. *Tailored Rehabilitation Plans:* A rehabilitation plan should be tailored to your specific needs, taking into account your treatment, surgery, and any pre-existing conditions. A physical therapist will assess your condition and create a personalized plan that aligns with your goals and limitations. Be open about your pain levels and any discomfort to ensure the plan is safe and effective.

6. *Commitment and Consistency*: Rehabilitation and physical therapy require commitment and consistency. Regular sessions with a physical therapist, along with exercises to do at home, are essential for a successful recovery. Follow the therapist's recommendations and be patient with your progress. Recovery is a journey that takes time.

7. *Additional Rehabilitation Services:* Rehabilitation may also include other services, such as occupational therapy, which focuses on daily activities and self-care, and speech therapy, if needed. Discuss with your healthcare team which services would be beneficial for you based on your specific condition and treatment.

8. *Monitoring Progress:* Your physical therapist will monitor your progress during rehabilitation. If you experience pain, increased fatigue, or other issues, communicate with your therapist to adjust the exercises or techniques as needed.

Regular monitoring ensures that you're on track to achieve your rehabilitation goals.

Rehabilitation and physical therapy can be transformative in your recovery after colorectal cancer treatment. By engaging in tailored exercises and being consistent with your therapy, you can improve your strength, mobility, and overall well-being. Remember to work closely with your healthcare team to ensure a safe and effective rehabilitation process.

Coping with Long-Term Side Effects

After completing treatment for colorectal cancer, many survivors face long-term side effects that can persist for months or even years. These effects can impact your quality of life and require ongoing management. Here's how you can cope with long-term side effects and find ways to improve your well-being.

1. Understanding Long-Term Side Effects: Long-term side effects can result from surgery, chemotherapy, radiation therapy, or other treatments. Common issues include:

- **Fatigue**: Persistent tiredness that can make it difficult to engage in daily activities.

- **Digestive Problems**: Changes in bowel habits, including diarrhea, constipation, or incontinence.

- **Peripheral Neuropathy**: Numbness, tingling, or pain in the hands and feet, often caused by chemotherapy.

- **Sexual Health Issues**: Changes in libido or sexual function due to treatment or emotional stress.

- **Emotional Challenges**: Anxiety, depression, or fear of recurrence.

2. Seek Support from Your Healthcare Team: Your healthcare team is your best resource for managing long-term side effects. They can help you understand the cause of your symptoms and recommend appropriate treatments or therapies. Regular follow-up appointments are crucial for monitoring your condition and addressing any ongoing issues.

3. Manage Fatigue: Fatigue can be a persistent challenge for colorectal cancer survivors. To manage fatigue:

- **Pace Yourself**: Spread out tasks throughout the day and take breaks when needed.

- **Exercise Regularly**: Light to moderate exercise, like walking or swimming, can boost energy levels.

- **Prioritize Sleep:** Aim for consistent sleep patterns and avoid caffeine or electronics before bedtime.

4. Address Digestive Problems: Digestive issues are common after colorectal cancer treatment. To manage these problems:

- **Adjust Your Diet**: A balanced diet with high-fiber foods can help with constipation, while low-fiber foods might be better for diarrhea. Drink plenty of water to stay hydrated.

- **Medications**: Your doctor may prescribe medications to manage specific digestive issues.

- **Work with a Dietitian:** A registered dietitian can help create a meal plan that suits your needs.

5. Manage Peripheral Neuropathy: Peripheral neuropathy can cause discomfort and affect your ability to perform daily tasks. To cope with neuropathy:

- **Physical Therapy**: Exercises to improve strength and coordination can be helpful.

- **Pain Management:** Medications or alternative therapies like acupuncture may relieve neuropathic pain.

- **Protect Your Hands and Feet**: Wear comfortable shoes and avoid activities that might cause injury due to numbness.

6. Address Sexual Health Issues: Changes in sexual health can be a sensitive topic but are important to address. To manage sexual health issues:

- **Open Communication**: Talk to your partner about your concerns and explore different forms of intimacy.

- **Seek Professional Help**: A therapist or counselor specializing in sexual health can offer guidance.

- **Explore Medical Options**: Medications or other treatments might be recommended by your healthcare provider.

7. *Tackle Emotional Challenges*: Emotional challenges can persist long after treatment ends. To cope with anxiety, depression, or fear of recurrence:

- **Seek Counseling:** A professional counselor can help you navigate complex emotions.

- **Join Support Groups**: Connecting with other survivors can provide comfort and reduce feelings of isolation.

- **Practice Relaxation Techniques**: Meditation, mindfulness, or yoga can help reduce stress and anxiety.

Coping with long-term side effects after colorectal cancer treatment requires patience and ongoing effort. By working closely with your healthcare team and using these strategies, you can manage these effects and focus on improving your quality of life.

Returning to Work and Normal Activities

Returning to work and resuming normal activities after colorectal cancer treatment is a significant milestone. It marks a step towards reclaiming your life and re-engaging with everyday routines. However, this transition can also be challenging, as it involves physical, emotional, and logistical considerations. Here's how to approach this process and what to keep in mind as you re-enter the workforce and other aspects of daily life.

1. Assess Your Readiness to Return to Work: Before returning to work, assess your physical and emotional readiness. Consider factors such as energy levels, treatment-related side effects, and any ongoing medical care. Speak with your healthcare team about your job's demands and whether you're ready to meet them. They can guide you on a suitable timeline for returning to work and suggest accommodations if needed.

2. Plan for a Gradual Return: A gradual return to work can be helpful if you're not ready for a full-time schedule. Discuss with your employer the possibility of a phased approach, such as reduced hours, part-time work, or a flexible schedule. This allows you to ease back into your role and adjust as needed.

3. Communicate with Your Employer: Open communication with your employer is essential when returning to work.

Inform them of any limitations or accommodations you might need, such as modified duties, extra breaks, or remote work. If you're unsure about your rights, refer to workplace laws like the Americans with Disabilities Act (ADA) or the Family and Medical Leave Act (FMLA) to understand what accommodations you're entitled to.

4. *Take Care of Your Health*: Returning to work can be physically and mentally demanding, so it's crucial to prioritize your health. Ensure you're getting enough rest, eating well, and staying active. If you experience fatigue or other side effects, find ways to manage them, such as taking breaks or adjusting your work environment.

5. *Reconnect with Colleagues and Social Activities*: Returning to work isn't just about the job—it's also about reconnecting with colleagues and resuming social activities. Take the time to catch up with co-workers and rebuild relationships. Social interactions can boost your mood and help you feel more integrated into the workplace.

6. *Set Boundaries and Manage Stress*: Returning to work after cancer treatment can be stressful. Set boundaries to avoid overexerting yourself. Learn to say no when necessary, and take time to relax and recharge. If work-related stress becomes overwhelming, consider talking to a counselor or therapist for additional support.

7. *Embrace Flexibility:* Flexibility is key when transitioning back to work. Be open to adjusting your schedule or duties as needed. If you find that certain tasks are too physically demanding or stressful, discuss alternatives with your employer. Flexibility can help you balance work and health more effectively.

8. *Celebrate Your Progress*: Returning to work and normal activities is a significant achievement. Celebrate your progress and acknowledge the effort it took to reach this point. Whether it's treating yourself to something special or sharing your success with friends and family, take time to recognize your accomplishments.

Returning to work and resuming normal activities after colorectal cancer requires careful planning and ongoing support. By communicating with your employer, setting boundaries, and taking care of your health, you can successfully navigate this transition and find a new balance in your life. Remember, it's okay to adjust at your own pace and seek help when needed. Your health and well-being should always come first.

Chapter 6: Living Well with Colorectal Cancer

Lifestyle Changes for Prevention and Management

Lifestyle choices can play a significant role in both the prevention and management of colorectal cancer. Making healthy changes can reduce the risk of developing the disease and improve outcomes for those already diagnosed. Some key lifestyle changes to consider for preventing and managing colorectal cancer.

1. Adopt a Healthy Diet: Diet is crucial in colorectal cancer prevention and management. Focus on eating a balanced diet rich in fruits, vegetables, whole grains, and lean proteins. Reduce the intake of red and processed meats, as they are linked to an increased risk of colorectal cancer. Instead, opt for fish, poultry, beans, and tofu as protein sources.

2. Maintain a Healthy Weight: Being overweight or obese increases the risk of colorectal cancer and can complicate treatment and recovery. Aim for a healthy weight through a combination of balanced nutrition and regular physical activity. Consult a healthcare provider or registered dietitian to determine your ideal weight and develop a plan to achieve it.

3. Stay Physically Active: Regular exercise has been proven to reduce the risk of colorectal cancer and enhance treatment outcomes. Strive for at least 30 minutes of moderate physical activity on most days. Walking, swimming, cycling, and yoga are great options. If you're new to exercising, begin slowly and gradually raise your activity level.

4. *Limit Alcohol Consumption:* Excessive alcohol consumption is associated with an increased risk of colorectal cancer. Limit alcohol to one drink per day for women and two drinks per day for men, or consider abstaining altogether. If you struggle to cut back on alcohol, seek help from a healthcare professional or counselor.

5. *Quit Smoking:* Smoking is a significant risk factor for many cancers, including colorectal cancer. If you smoke, quitting is one of the most beneficial actions you can take for your health. There are various resources available to help you quit smoking, including nicotine replacement therapy, counseling, and support groups.

6. *Manage Stress:* Chronic stress can negatively impact your health and weaken your immune system. Find healthy ways to manage stress, such as meditation, mindfulness, deep breathing exercises, or spending time in nature. Regular physical activity and engaging in hobbies you enjoy can also help reduce stress levels.

7. Get Regular Screenings: Regular screenings are crucial for early detection and prevention of colorectal cancer. Follow your healthcare provider's recommendations for colonoscopies and other screening tests based on your age, family history, and other risk factors. Detecting conditions early can greatly enhance treatment results.

8. Build a Support Network: Having a strong support network can make a significant difference in managing colorectal cancer. Connect with family, friends, support groups, and healthcare professionals for emotional support and guidance. These connections can help you navigate challenges and maintain a positive outlook.

9. Prioritize Sleep and Rest: Adequate sleep is essential for overall health and well-being. Aim for 7 to 9 hours of sleep per night and establish a consistent sleep routine. If you have trouble sleeping, try relaxation techniques or create a calming bedtime environment.

10. Stay Informed and Advocate for Your Health: Knowledge is power when it comes to managing colorectal cancer. Keep yourself educated about your condition, treatment choices, and the latest research. Feel free to ask questions or seek a second opinion if necessary. Advocate for your health and work collaboratively with your healthcare team.

By making these lifestyle changes, you can reduce the risk of colorectal cancer and improve your overall health. These changes are beneficial not only for prevention but also for managing the disease and supporting recovery. Take small steps toward a healthier lifestyle, and remember that each positive change can have a lasting impact on your well-being.

Nutritional Guidelines for Survivorship

Nutrition plays a vital role in the recovery and long-term health of colorectal cancer survivors. Adopting a balanced diet can help boost energy, maintain a healthy weight, and reduce the risk of cancer recurrence. These nutritional guidelines provide a clear approach to eating well during survivorship.

1. *Focus on a Plant-Based Diet:* A diet rich in plant-based foods can offer numerous health benefits. Aim to fill your plate with a variety of fruits, vegetables, whole grains, and legumes. These foods are high in fiber, vitamins, minerals, and antioxidants, all of which contribute to overall health.

2. *Choose Lean Proteins*: Include lean sources of protein in your diet to support muscle repair and overall energy. Good options include chicken, fish, turkey, eggs, tofu, beans, and low-fat dairy products. Limit red and processed meats, as these have been linked to an increased risk of colorectal cancer.

3. *Limit Added Sugars and Processed Foods:* Cut back on foods with high levels of added sugars, such as sugary drinks, desserts, and candies. Processed foods often contain unhealthy

fats and preservatives. Instead, choose whole, unprocessed foods whenever possible. Natural sweeteners like honey or maple syrup can be used in moderation.

4. *Include Healthy Fats:* Healthy fats are important for heart health and can be found in foods like avocados, nuts, seeds, and olive oil. Incorporate these into your diet, but avoid trans fats and limit saturated fats, typically found in fried foods and high-fat dairy products.

5. *Stay Hydrated:* Proper hydration is crucial for health, especially during and after cancer treatment. Make it a goal to stay well-hydrated by drinking plenty of water throughout the day. Herbal teas and flavored water (without added sugars) are also good options. Limit caffeine and alcohol, as they can lead to dehydration and other health issues.

6. *Control Portion Sizes:* Maintaining a healthy weight is key to reducing the risk of cancer recurrence. To avoid overeating, concentrate on managing portion sizes. Use smaller plates, and avoid eating straight from packages. Pay attention to your body and stop eating when you feel full.

7. *Practice Mindful Eating:* Mindful eating involves paying attention to the food you eat and enjoying each bite. Slow down, savor your meals, and avoid distractions like television or smartphones during mealtimes. This practice can help you connect with your food and make healthier choices.

8. *Monitor for Food Sensitivities*: Some colorectal cancer survivors may develop food sensitivities or digestive issues after treatment. If you experience discomfort or digestive problems after eating certain foods, keep a food journal to identify potential triggers. Discuss any concerns with a registered dietitian or your healthcare provider.

9. Consult a Registered Dietitian: A registered dietitian with experience in cancer survivorship can offer personalized nutritional advice. They can help you create a balanced meal plan that suits your preferences and addresses any specific dietary needs.

10. Balance Nutrition with Physical Activity: A healthy diet is just one part of the survivorship equation. Combine it with regular physical activity to maintain muscle mass, boost energy, and support your overall well-being. Find activities you enjoy and incorporate them into your routine.

Following these nutritional guidelines can help you maintain a healthy lifestyle and reduce the risk of cancer recurrence. As you navigate survivorship, remember that good nutrition is a journey, not a destination. Experiment with different foods, find what works best for you, and enjoy the process of discovering new flavors and meals that support your health.

Exercise and Physical Activity Recommendations

Staying active during colorectal cancer treatment and recovery can improve your physical health, boost your mood, and help you manage treatment side effects. Exercise doesn't have to be intense or lengthy—even light activity can make a significant difference. The following recommendations will help you incorporate exercise and physical activity into your routine safely and effectively.

1. Start Slowly and Listen to Your Body: Begin with light activities, especially if you're new to exercise or recovering from surgery. Walking, stretching, or gentle yoga are good starting points. Pay attention to how your body responds to activity and adjust your pace accordingly. If you feel pain or discomfort, stop and rest. Always consult your healthcare team before starting a new exercise regimen.

2. Aim for Consistency: Consistency is key to reaping the benefits of exercise. Aim for regular activity, even if it's just a short walk each day. Consistency helps improve energy levels, maintain muscle mass, and enhance overall well-being. Find a time that works best for you—morning, afternoon, or evening—and stick to it.

3. Incorporate Different Types of Exercise: A varied exercise routine can keep things interesting and target different aspects of fitness. Consider including the following types of exercise:

- **Aerobic Exercise:** Activities like walking, swimming, or cycling can improve cardiovascular health and boost energy levels. Aim for at least 30 minutes of moderate aerobic activity most days, if possible.

- **Strength Training**: Using light weights or resistance bands can help maintain muscle strength. Focus on exercises that target major muscle groups, such as biceps, triceps, chest, back, and legs.

- **Flexibility and Balance**: Activities like yoga, tai chi, or simple stretching can improve flexibility, balance, and coordination. These exercises can also help reduce stress and improve mental clarity.

4. Exercise with Others: Exercising with a friend, family member, or group can make physical activity more enjoyable and help you stay motivated. Consider joining a fitness class designed for cancer patients, or find a walking or exercise buddy to keep you company. Group activities provide social support, which is beneficial during cancer treatment.

5. Adjust for Treatment Side Effects: Cancer treatment can cause fatigue, nausea, and other side effects that affect your ability to exercise. Adjust your routine to accommodate these challenges. If you're fatigued, try shorter sessions or lower-intensity exercises. If nausea is an issue, focus on deep breathing and relaxation techniques before exercising. Discuss any persistent side effects with your healthcare team.

6. Prioritize Safety: Safety is crucial when incorporating exercise and physical activity into your routine. Follow these safety tips:

- **Warm-Up and Cool-Down**: Always warm up before exercise and cool down afterward to prevent injury and ease into physical activity.

- **Stay Hydrated:** Drink plenty of water before, during, and after exercise to stay hydrated.

- **Wear Appropriate Clothing**: Choose comfortable, breathable clothing and proper footwear to avoid discomfort or injury.

7. Focus on Enjoyment: Exercise should be enjoyable, not a chore. Find activities that you like and that fit your interests. Whether it's dancing, gardening, or playing with pets, focus on what brings you joy while keeping you active.

Exercise and physical activity can play a vital role in your colorectal cancer journey. By starting slowly, aiming for consistency, and focusing on different types of exercise, you can improve your health and well-being during treatment and recovery. Always consult your healthcare team before beginning any exercise routine to ensure it's safe and suitable for your specific needs.

Stress Management and Mental Well-Being

A diagnosis of colorectal cancer can lead to significant stress, anxiety, and emotional upheaval. Managing stress and maintaining mental well-being are crucial as you undergo treatment and navigate the changes it brings to your life. Below are ways to help you cope with stress and foster mental well-being during colorectal cancer treatment:

1. Understand the Sources of Stress: Colorectal cancer treatment can introduce various sources of stress, such as:

- **Uncertainty**: Concerns about treatment outcomes and future health.

- **Physical Discomfort:** Pain, fatigue, or other side effects from treatment.

- **Lifestyle Changes**: Disruptions to work, family, and social life.

- **Emotional Impact:** Feelings of sadness, fear, or anger.

Acknowledging these sources of stress is the first step in managing them effectively.

2. Establish a Support System: A strong support system can make a significant difference in your ability to cope with stress. Consider the following sources of support:

- **Family and Friends:** Share your feelings with those close to you. Let them know how best they can support you.

- **Support Groups**: Connecting with others who are going through similar experiences can provide comfort and valuable insights.

- **Counselors or Therapists**: Professional guidance from mental health experts can be invaluable in managing stress and emotional challenges.

3. Practice Relaxation Techniques: Relaxation techniques can help you manage stress and improve mental well-being. Some popular techniques include:

- **Deep Breathing**: Focused breathing exercises can reduce stress and promote relaxation.

- **Meditation**: Meditation and mindfulness practices help you stay grounded and present in the moment.

- **Yoga or Tai Chi:** Gentle exercises that combine physical movement with mindfulness can be calming.

4. Maintain a Healthy Lifestyle: A healthy lifestyle can support your mental well-being and reduce stress. Aim to:

- **Exercise Regularly**: Even light physical activity, like walking or stretching, can boost mood and reduce stress.

- Eat **Nutritious Foods**: A balanced diet helps keep your energy levels up and supports overall health.

- **Get Adequate Sleep**: Good sleep is crucial for mental and physical recovery. Establish a regular sleep routine and create a comfortable sleeping environment.

5. Set Realistic Expectations: Colorectal cancer treatment is a journey with ups and downs. Set realistic expectations for yourself and understand that it's okay to have difficult days. Give yourself permission to feel a range of emotions without judgment.

6. Stay Connected with Your Healthcare Team: Your healthcare team is not only there to guide your medical treatment but also to support your mental well-being. If you're struggling with stress or emotional issues, discuss them with your team. They can recommend resources and connect you with professionals who can help.

7. Find Activities That Bring Joy: Engage in activities that bring you joy and relaxation. This might include hobbies, spending time with loved ones, listening to music, or exploring nature. Doing things you enjoy can be a great way to relieve stress and boost your mood.

8. Limit Negative Influences: Be mindful of sources that can increase stress, such as negative news or unsupportive people. Limit exposure to these influences, and focus on positive, uplifting environments.

Managing stress and maintaining mental well-being during colorectal cancer treatment is a continuous process. By building a strong support system, practicing relaxation techniques, and leading a healthy lifestyle, you can better cope with the emotional challenges and focus on your recovery and overall quality of life.

Sexual Health and Intimacy

Colorectal cancer treatment can impact various aspects of your life, including sexual health and intimacy. It's important to understand that changes in sexual desire, performance, or intimacy are common during treatment. Things you need to know about maintaining sexual health and intimacy during colorectal cancer treatment:

1. Recognize Common Changes: Treatment for colorectal cancer can lead to physical and emotional changes that affect sexual health. Some common changes include:

- **Reduced Libido**: Fatigue, stress, and treatment side effects can decrease sexual desire.

- **Physical Discomfort**: Pain, scarring, or other physical issues may make intimacy challenging.

- **Emotional Impact:** Anxiety, depression, or body image concerns can affect intimacy.

These changes are normal, and many people experience them during cancer treatment.

2. Communicate with Your Partner: Open communication with your partner is crucial for maintaining intimacy. Talk about your feelings, fears, and concerns related to sexual health. Discuss how you can both adapt to changes and support each other through the treatment process.

3. Explore Different Forms of Intimacy: Intimacy isn't limited to sexual activity. Explore other ways to connect with your partner, such as:

- **Emotional Intimacy**: Share your thoughts and feelings openly.

- **Physical Affection**: Hold hands, hug, or cuddle to maintain closeness.

- **Shared Activities:** Engage in activities you both enjoy to strengthen your bond.

These forms of intimacy can help maintain a strong connection even if sexual activity is limited.

4. Manage Physical Discomfort: If you're experiencing physical discomfort during intimacy, consider these tips:

- **Positioning**: Experiment with different positions to find what's comfortable.

- **Lubrication**: If vaginal dryness is an issue, use water-based lubricants to reduce discomfort.

- **Timing**: Choose times when you're feeling rested and less fatigued.

Discuss any persistent pain or discomfort with your healthcare team to identify possible solutions.

5. Address Emotional Concerns: Emotional issues can significantly impact sexual health and intimacy. If you're feeling anxious, depressed, or struggling with body image concerns, consider seeking support from a counselor or therapist. Professional support can help you work through these emotions and improve your overall well-being.

6. Understand the Impact of Medications: Some medications used in colorectal cancer treatment can affect sexual health. Chemotherapy and hormone therapy can cause hormonal changes that reduce libido. If you suspect your medication is affecting your sexual health, discuss it with your doctor. They may be able to adjust your medication or offer other solutions.

7. Be Patient with Yourself: Recovery from colorectal cancer and its treatment takes time, and it's normal for sexual health and intimacy to fluctuate during this period. Be patient with yourself and your partner as you navigate these changes. Remember that rebuilding intimacy is a journey, not a race.

8. Seek Professional Guidance: If you're struggling with sexual health and intimacy, consider speaking with a healthcare professional who specializes in sexual health or oncology-related intimacy issues. They can provide advice, therapy, or medical solutions tailored to your needs.

Sexual health and intimacy are important aspects of quality of life. By maintaining open communication, exploring different forms of intimacy, and seeking professional support when needed, you can navigate the challenges of colorectal cancer treatment and find meaningful ways to connect with your partner.

Chapter 7: Resources and Support

Finding Reliable Information and Resources

When you're diagnosed with colorectal cancer, one of the first things you might do is search for information. It's crucial to find accurate, reliable resources to guide you through your treatment and recovery. Here's how you can identify trustworthy sources and make the best use of the information available:

1. Start with Your Healthcare Team: Your healthcare team is the most reliable source of information about your diagnosis, treatment options, and follow-up care. Don't hesitate to ask questions and seek clarification about anything you're unsure of. They can also provide brochures, pamphlets, and other educational materials to help you understand your condition.

2. Use Reputable Medical Websites: Several reputable websites offer reliable information about colorectal cancer. These websites are generally associated with well-known medical institutions, cancer organizations, or government agencies. Here are a few trusted sources:

- American Cancer Society (ACS): Offers detailed information on colorectal cancer, including treatment, side effects, and support resources.

- National Cancer Institute (NCI): Provides comprehensive information on various cancer types, including clinical trials and cancer research.

- Cancer Research UK: Offers patient-friendly information and resources, especially for those in the UK.

Ensure that the information you find on these websites is up-to-date and backed by scientific evidence.

3. Be Cautious with Personal Blogs and Forums: While personal blogs and online forums can be a source of support and shared experiences, they may not always contain accurate or reliable information. Use these platforms to connect with others, but double-check any medical advice or treatment suggestions with your healthcare team.

4. Seek Recommendations from Cancer Support Organizations: Cancer support organizations often offer resources tailored to cancer patients and their families. They can connect you with support groups, counseling services, and financial assistance programs. Some well-known cancer support organizations include:

- CancerCare: Provides free counseling, support groups, and educational resources for cancer patients and caregivers.

- The American Society of Clinical Oncology (ASCO): Offers educational resources and expert advice for patients.

- Colorectal Cancer Alliance: A nonprofit organization focused on colorectal cancer, providing support, education, and advocacy.

5. *Look for Peer-Reviewed Information*: Peer-reviewed information has been evaluated by other experts in the field, indicating that it meets certain standards of accuracy and quality. Scientific journals and research publications often contain peer-reviewed information, which can be a reliable source for deeper insights into colorectal cancer.

6. *Be Skeptical of Quick Fixes and "Miracle" Cures*: If a source promises a quick fix, miracle cure, or claims to have information that "doctors don't want you to know," it's likely unreliable. Reliable sources focus on evidence-based treatment options and do not make unrealistic promises.

7. *Stay Informed but Avoid Overwhelm*: While it's important to stay informed, reading too much information at once can be overwhelming. Focus on learning what you need to know about your diagnosis, treatment, and next steps. If you feel stressed or confused by the information, take a break and discuss your concerns with your healthcare team.

Finding reliable information and resources is key to navigating your colorectal cancer journey. By using reputable websites, seeking advice from your healthcare team, and staying cautious of unreliable sources, you can ensure you're making informed decisions about your treatment and care.

Financial Assistance and Insurance

A diagnosis of colorectal cancer can lead to significant financial concerns. From treatment costs to time off work, the financial impact can be substantial. Things you need to know about managing financial challenges and navigating insurance when dealing with colorectal cancer:

1. Understanding Treatment Costs: Colorectal cancer treatment can be expensive, involving costs for:

- **Medical Appointments**: Including consultations with doctors and specialists.

- **Diagnostic Tests:** Scans, biopsies, and other tests to diagnose and monitor the cancer.

- **Treatment**: Surgery, chemotherapy, radiation therapy, and other treatments.

- **Medications**: Prescription drugs to manage side effects or prevent recurrence.

- **Hospital Stays**: If surgery or other treatment requires hospitalization.

Knowing the potential costs can help you plan and find the right resources to manage them.

2. Review Your Insurance Coverage: Insurance can play a significant role in offsetting medical costs. Here are some key steps to ensure you're maximizing your coverage:

- **Understand Your Policy:** Review your insurance policy to understand what is covered and what is not. Pay attention to deductibles, copayments, and out-of-pocket maximums.

- **Work with an Insurance Specialist**: Some hospitals have patient navigators or financial counselors who can help you understand your insurance benefits and advocate for coverage.

- **Get Pre-Authorizations**: Before undergoing expensive procedures or treatments, check whether pre-authorization is needed to ensure coverage.

3. Financial Assistance Programs: If you're facing financial challenges, consider these resources for assistance:

- **Government Programs:** Programs like Medicaid, Medicare, or Supplemental Security Income (SSI) may be available depending on your eligibility.

- **Nonprofit Organizations**: Several organizations offer financial assistance for cancer patients, including help with medical bills, transportation, and other needs. Examples include the CancerCare Co-Payment Assistance Foundation and the HealthWell Foundation.

- **Hospital Assistance Programs**: Some hospitals have financial assistance programs for uninsured or underinsured patients. Ask your hospital's billing department about these programs.

- **Patient Assistance Programs:** Certain pharmaceutical companies offer assistance for expensive medications. Check with your doctor or nurse about these programs.

4. Consider Legal Protections: Laws such as the Americans with Disabilities Act (ADA) and the Family and Medical Leave Act (FMLA) provide protections for cancer patients. These laws can help ensure job security and reasonable accommodations during treatment and recovery.

5. Budget and Plan Ahead: Creating a budget can help you manage the financial impact of cancer treatment. Consider:

- **Tracking Expenses**: Keep a record of all medical-related costs, including transportation, parking, and meals during treatment.

- **Reducing Non-Essential Spending**: Focus on necessities and cut back on non-essential expenses to reduce financial stress.

- **Seeking Advice**: A financial advisor or counselor can help you create a budget and plan for future expenses.

6. *Explore Fundraising Options:* If you need additional financial support, consider fundraising options. Crowdfunding platforms like GoFundMe can help you raise money from family, friends, and the community. However, approach fundraising with sensitivity and clarity about your needs.

7. *Utilize Community Resources*: Local community organizations and charities may offer support for cancer patients. This can include transportation services, meal deliveries, or financial assistance for specific needs. Check with local cancer support groups or community centers for available resources.

Financial assistance and insurance support are critical when dealing with colorectal cancer. By understanding your insurance coverage, exploring financial assistance programs, and planning your budget, you can reduce financial stress and focus on your treatment and recovery. If you need additional guidance, consider reaching out to a financial counselor or patient advocate for personalized support.

Legal Rights and Advocacy

A colorectal cancer diagnosis often leads to numerous questions about your legal rights, from workplace accommodations to medical privacy. Understanding your legal rights can help you navigate the complexities of cancer treatment and ensure you're treated fairly. Here's what you need to know about your legal rights and advocacy as a colorectal cancer patient:

1. Workplace Rights and Protections: A colorectal cancer diagnosis can impact your ability to work. However, there are legal protections to ensure you are treated fairly in the workplace:

- **Americans with Disabilities Act (ADA):** This law prohibits discrimination against people with disabilities, including those with cancer. Under the ADA, employers must provide reasonable accommodations, such as flexible work hours or modifications to your workspace, unless it causes undue hardship.

- **Family and Medical Leave Act (FMLA):** FMLA provides eligible employees with up to 12 weeks of unpaid leave per year for serious health conditions, including cancer. This leave can be utilized for treatment, recovery, or caring for a family member with a serious health condition.

- **Equal Employment Opportunity**: Laws ensure that you cannot be fired or discriminated against because of your cancer diagnosis or treatment. If you feel your rights are being violated, you can file a complaint with the Equal Employment Opportunity Commission (EEOC).

2. *Health Insurance Rights:* Health insurance laws protect your access to coverage and prevent discrimination based on your cancer diagnosis:

- **Affordable Care Act (ACA):** The ACA prohibits health insurance companies from denying coverage due to pre-existing conditions like cancer. It also requires most health plans to cover essential health benefits, including cancer treatment.

- **COBRA**: If you lose your job, the Consolidated Omnibus Budget Reconciliation Act (COBRA) allows you to continue your employer-provided health insurance for a limited time, usually at your own expense.

- **HIPAA**: The Health Insurance Portability and Accountability Act (HIPAA) ensures that your medical information is kept private. Healthcare providers must obtain your consent to share your medical information with others, ensuring your privacy during treatment.

3. Medical Decision-Making Rights: As a colorectal cancer patient, you have the right to make informed decisions about your treatment:

- **Informed Consent:** Before any medical procedure, you have the right to understand the risks, benefits, and alternatives. Your healthcare provider must explain this information clearly, allowing you to make informed decisions.

- **Advance Directives:** These legal documents allow you to express your wishes regarding medical treatment if you become unable to make decisions. Common advance directives include living wills and durable powers of attorney for healthcare.

4. Advocacy and Support: Advocacy organizations can provide guidance and support on legal rights and related issues:

- **Patient Advocates:** Many hospitals have patient advocates who can help you navigate the healthcare system, resolve conflicts, and ensure your rights are upheld.

- **Cancer Advocacy Organizations**: Organizations like the American Cancer Society and the Colorectal Cancer Alliance offer resources and legal support for cancer patients.

- **Legal Aid Services:** If you need legal assistance but cannot afford a lawyer, consider contacting legal aid services or nonprofit organizations that specialize in healthcare-related legal issues.

5. *Know Your Rights and Seek Help*: Understanding your legal rights and advocacy options is essential when dealing with colorectal cancer. If you're unsure about your rights or need help with a legal issue, seek advice from a lawyer specializing in healthcare law or employee rights. Many cancer advocacy organizations offer legal resources and can guide you in the right direction.

Legal rights and advocacy are crucial to protecting your interests and ensuring fair treatment during colorectal cancer treatment. By knowing your rights and seeking support from patient advocates and legal experts, you can focus on your health and recovery without unnecessary stress or discrimination.

Additional Support Services

Navigating a colorectal cancer diagnosis can be overwhelming. While medical treatment is a significant focus, other aspects of your life also require support. Additional support services are available to help you manage the practical, emotional, and financial challenges that come with cancer. Here's an overview of the support services that may be beneficial to you:

1. Transportation Assistance: Getting to and from medical appointments can be challenging, especially during treatment when fatigue or other side effects are prevalent. Some organizations offer transportation services to help you with this:
- **American Cancer Society's Road to Recovery**: This program provides volunteer drivers to transport cancer patients to treatment appointments.
- **Local Nonprofits and Community Programs**: Check for local programs that offer free or low-cost transportation to medical appointments.

2. Meal Delivery Services: Preparing meals can be difficult during cancer treatment. Meal delivery services can help ensure you have nutritious meals without the stress of cooking:
- **Meals on Wheels**: This service delivers meals to individuals who need assistance with meal preparation.
- **Community and Religious Organizations**: Some local groups offer meal delivery or meal train services to support those undergoing cancer treatment.

3. Child Care Assistance: If you have children, arranging childcare during medical appointments or treatment can be challenging. Some organizations offer childcare support for cancer patients:

- **Cancer Support Organizations**: Check with cancer support organizations for programs that offer child care or assistance finding childcare services.

- **Local Community Resources**: Community centers, religious groups, or local nonprofits may offer childcare services or connect you with providers.

4. *Financial Counseling:* Cancer treatment can lead to financial strain. Financial counseling services can help you manage costs and explore financial assistance options:

- **Hospital Financial Counselors:** Many hospitals have financial counselors to help you understand your medical bills, insurance coverage, and available assistance programs.
- **Nonprofit Financial Aid Programs**: Some organizations provide grants or assistance to cancer patients to cover medical bills, transportation, or other expenses.

5. *Career and Employment Support:* Colorectal cancer can impact your ability to work or pursue career goals. Employment support services can help you navigate workplace issues and make necessary accommodations:

- **Job Accommodation Network (JAN):** This organization offers guidance on workplace accommodations and employment rights for people with disabilities, including cancer patients.
- **Vocational Rehabilitation Services**: State-run programs can help you find new employment opportunities or retrain for different roles if needed.

6. *Pet Care Services*: If you have pets, arranging their care during treatment or hospital stays can be a concern. Some organizations offer pet care support for cancer patients:

- **Local Animal Shelters and Rescue Groups**: These organizations may offer temporary foster care or pet care assistance during your treatment.
- **Friends and Family**: Consider reaching out to loved ones for help with pet care during your treatment.

7. *Spiritual and Faith-Based Support:* Spiritual and faith-based support can provide comfort and guidance during difficult times. Seek out these resources if they align with your beliefs:

- **Hospital Chaplaincy Services:** Many hospitals offer chaplaincy services to support patients' spiritual needs.
- **Religious and Spiritual Communities**: Connect with local churches, temples, or other spiritual communities for support and counseling.

These additional support services can help alleviate the practical challenges that come with colorectal cancer. By utilizing transportation assistance, meal delivery, financial counseling, and other support resources, you can focus on your health and well-being during treatment and recovery. If you need more information about these services, ask your healthcare team or patient advocate for guidance and recommendations.

Chapter 8: Stories of Hope and Inspiration

Personal Stories from Survivors and Caregivers

1. John's Journey:

From Shock to Advocacy John, a 45-year-old father of two, received a colorectal cancer diagnosis after experiencing abdominal pain and changes in his bowel habits. "The moment the doctor said 'cancer,' I felt like the ground disappeared beneath me," he recalls. The shock was immediate, and fear took over. He worried about how he would explain the diagnosis to his children and how he could manage his job during treatment.

John's wife, Lisa, became his primary caregiver. She took on the role of researching treatment options, accompanying him to appointments, and coordinating with doctors. "It was a learning curve, but I wanted to make sure he had all the support he needed," Lisa says. Together, they navigated chemotherapy, surgery, and radiation therapy.

During treatment, John found solace in a local support group. "It was comforting to hear from others who had been through it," he says. "I wasn't alone, and that made a huge difference." The support group also gave Lisa a chance to connect with other caregivers, sharing tips and encouragement.

After completing treatment, John felt compelled to give back. He started volunteering with a cancer advocacy organization, sharing his story and raising awareness about the importance of early detection. "I want people to know that you can get through this," he says. "It's not easy, but there's life after cancer."

2. Maria's Recovery:

Finding Strength in Family Maria, a 63-year-old grandmother, faced her colorectal cancer diagnosis with a mix of fear and determination. "I knew I had to fight," she recalls. "I had too much to live for—my children, my grandchildren. I wasn't ready to give up."

Her treatment plan included surgery followed by chemotherapy. The surgery was successful, but the recovery was longer than expected. "I couldn't move around much, and I needed help with the simplest things," she says. Her family stepped in, with her daughter, Anna, taking time off work to care for her. "Anna was amazing," Maria says. "She cooked, cleaned, and made sure I took my medication on time."

Chemotherapy brought new challenges—nausea, fatigue, and hair loss. But Maria's grandchildren became her motivation. "They'd come over and sit with me, bring me drawings, and just make me smile," she says. "It gave me the strength to keep going."

After treatment, Maria focused on rebuilding her strength and finding a new normal. She started walking in the park every day, gradually increasing her distance. "It was a slow process, but each step felt like progress," she says. Her advice to others? "Don't rush yourself. Recovery takes time, and it's perfectly fine to rely on others for support."

3. Steve's Story:

Overcoming the Fear of Recurrence Steve, a 55-year-old teacher, successfully completed treatment for colorectal cancer, but the fear of recurrence lingered. "Every little pain or discomfort made me worry," he admits. "It felt like the cancer was always lurking in the background."

He decided to address his fears by focusing on his health. Steve adopted a healthier diet, started exercising regularly, and joined a mindfulness meditation class. "It helped me calm my mind and focus on the present," he says. "I stopped letting fear control me."

Steve's wife, Karen, supported him through this journey. "We spent a lot of time together—cooking healthy meals, taking walks, and practicing meditation," she says. "It wasn't just about physical health; it was about emotional healing too."

Steve also found support in a cancer survivor group. "Talking to others who'd been through it helped me realize I wasn't the only one feeling this way," he says. The group shared tips on managing anxiety and maintaining a positive outlook.

Today, Steve continues to focus on his health and encourages others to do the same. "Take care of your physical and mental well-being," he advises. "Surround yourself with positive people and engage in activities that bring you joy". It makes a difference."

Overcoming Challenges and Finding Strength

A colorectal cancer diagnosis brings many challenges—physical, emotional, and practical. While these hurdles may seem overwhelming, many people find strength in unexpected places and discover new sources of resilience. Here are some ways to overcome the challenges of colorectal cancer and find the strength to move forward:

1. Embrace a Positive Mindset: Maintaining a positive outlook can be challenging, especially during difficult times. However, focusing on hope and the possibility of recovery can make a big difference in your journey. Try these approaches to cultivate a positive mindset:

- **Practice Gratitude**: Identify and appreciate the good things in your life, no matter how small.

- **Set Achievable Goals:** Break down large tasks into smaller, manageable steps, and celebrate your progress.

- **Seek Inspirational Stories**: Hearing about others who have overcome similar challenges can provide encouragement and motivation.

2. Build a Strong Support Network: Support from family, friends, healthcare providers, and support groups can provide emotional strength and practical assistance. Building a strong support network can help you navigate the journey with confidence:

- **Lean on Loved Ones**: Allow family and friends to help you with daily tasks, transportation, or simply to listen and offer emotional support.

- **Join a Support Group:** Connecting with others who are facing similar challenges can be comforting and provide valuable insights.

- **Communicate Openly**: Share your feelings and needs with those around you. This openness can strengthen your relationships and improve the support you receive.

3. Prioritize Self-Care: Taking care of your physical and mental well-being is crucial for overcoming challenges and finding strength. Focus on these key aspects of self-care:

- **Nutrition**: Eat a balanced diet rich in fruits, vegetables, and whole grains to support your health and energy levels.

- **Exercise**: Engage in physical activity that suits your condition and abilities, such as walking or gentle stretching.

- **Rest and Relaxation**: Prioritize sleep and find relaxation techniques that work for you, like deep breathing, meditation, or listening to soothing music.

4. Stay Informed and Involved: Understanding your diagnosis and treatment options can help you feel more in control and reduce anxiety. Engage with your healthcare team and stay informed about your condition:

- **Ask Questions**: Don't hesitate to ask your doctors and nurses about your treatment, side effects, and what to expect.

- **Research Trusted Sources**: Use reputable websites and resources to learn more about colorectal cancer and available treatments.
- **Participate in Your Care**: Be actively involved in decision-making and collaborate with your healthcare team to create a treatment plan that works for you.

5. Find Meaning and Purpose: Many people find strength in discovering new meaning and purpose during their cancer journey. This could involve connecting with your values, pursuing new interests, or giving back to others:

- **Reconnect with Your Passions**: Rediscover hobbies or activities that bring you joy and fulfillment.
- **Help Others:** Consider volunteering, participating in cancer awareness events, or supporting others going through similar experiences.
- **Focus on What Matters:** Take time to reflect on your values and what is truly important to you. This can help you navigate the challenges with clarity and determination.

6. Seek Professional Support: If you're struggling with the emotional and psychological aspects of colorectal cancer, seeking professional support can be beneficial:

- **Counseling or Therapy:** Speaking with a licensed therapist or counselor can help you process your emotions and develop coping strategies.
- **Medication for Anxiety or Depression**: If needed, your healthcare provider may recommend medication to help manage anxiety or depression.

Finding strength in the face of colorectal cancer is a deeply personal journey. By embracing a positive mindset, building a strong support network, prioritizing self-care, staying informed, finding meaning and purpose, and seeking professional support, you can overcome challenges and navigate the road ahead with resilience and courage.

Messages of Hope and Encouragement

A colorectal cancer diagnosis can be daunting, but it's important to remember that you are not alone. Many have walked this path before you, and their experiences show that there is hope, even in the midst of challenging times. Here are some messages of hope and encouragement to help you stay strong and positive as you navigate your journey:

1. You Are Stronger Than You Know: Colorectal cancer can test your limits, but you may find strength and resilience within yourself that you never knew existed. Take one step at a time, and know that each day you are making progress.

2. You Are Not Alone: Surround yourself with people who care about you. Lean on your family, friends, and healthcare team for support. There are many others who understand what you're going through, and they are ready to walk with you through the ups and downs.

3. Treatment Is Improving Every Day: Medical advancements in colorectal cancer treatment continue to improve outcomes. With new therapies, better technology, and innovative approaches, there is more hope than ever for a positive outcome. Trust in your medical team and stay informed about the latest treatment options.

4. Take Time to Celebrate Small Victories: Progress doesn't always come in big leaps. Sometimes it's the small victories that matter most. Whether it's completing a round of treatment, taking a walk around the block, or simply having a good day, take time to celebrate these moments. They are signs of your strength and resilience.

5. Keep a Positive Outlook: Staying positive can be challenging, but it can also make a big difference in how you experience your journey. Focus on what you can control and find joy in the things that make you happy. A positive mindset can be a powerful tool in your recovery.

6. It's Okay to Ask for Help: You don't have to do this alone. If you need help, ask for it. Whether it's a ride to the hospital, assistance with meals, or just someone to talk to, reaching out is a sign of strength, not weakness. People care about you and want to support you through this journey.

7. You Have the Power to Inspire Others: Your journey can be an inspiration to others. By facing challenges with courage and determination, you are showing others that they too can overcome adversity. Share your story, connect with other survivors, and be a beacon of hope for those who may need it.

8. There Is Life Beyond Cancer: While colorectal cancer is a significant chapter in your life, it's not the whole story. Many survivors go on to lead fulfilling, joyful lives after treatment. Keep dreaming, keep planning for the future, and remember that you have a lot to look forward to.

9. Trust Yourself and Your Body: You know yourself better than anyone. Trust your instincts, listen to your body, and communicate with your healthcare team about any concerns. Your health and well-being are the most important things, and you have the right to advocate for yourself.

10. Take Each Day as It Comes: Some days will be harder than others, but every day is a new opportunity. Embrace each day with an open heart and mind, and focus on the present. The future is uncertain, but by taking things one day at a time, you can find peace and strength.

These messages of hope and encouragement are reminders that, even in the face of colorectal cancer, you can find strength, support, and a path forward. Stay connected with those who care about you, maintain a positive outlook, and keep believing in your own resilience. You have what it takes to get through this, and you are not alone on this journey.

Conclusion

You've just learned a lot about colorectal cancer—what it is, the causes and risks, the treatment options, and how to navigate the emotional and practical challenges it brings. It's a lot to take in, and it's normal to feel a bit overwhelmed. But now, as we reach the end of this guide, I want you to remember one thing: you're not alone in this journey.

Whether you're at the beginning of treatment, in the middle of it, or moving into recovery, this journey is yours. It's okay to have questions, to feel uncertain, and to experience a range of emotions. What's most important is that you give yourself the space and grace to navigate this at your own pace.

Surround yourself with people who care about you. Lean on them when you need to, and don't hesitate to ask for help. The support you receive from family, friends, and healthcare professionals can make a world of difference. Find comfort in knowing that there's a community of survivors, caregivers, and medical experts who are here to support you.

As you look ahead, consider this an opportunity to redefine what life means to you. It might not be easy, and there will be days when it feels like too much. But each day you take a step forward, you're moving toward a future where colorectal cancer doesn't define you.

Remember to focus on your well-being. Eating well, staying active, and finding moments of joy are all crucial parts of your recovery. Don't forget to take care of your mental and emotional health too—talking to a counselor or joining a support group can be incredibly helpful.

I want to encourage you to hold onto hope. Hope is a powerful thing, and it can carry you through even the darkest times. Whether it's the hope of recovery, the hope of a future without cancer, or simply the hope of a good day, it's something worth holding onto.

Keep moving forward, keep believing in yourself, and never forget that you have a network of support ready to help you along the way. You've got this. We believe in you.

Appendices

Glossary of Terms

Adjuvant Therapy: Additional treatment given after the primary treatment to reduce the risk of cancer recurrence. This can include chemotherapy, radiation therapy, or targeted therapy.

Benign: A term used to describe a tumor or growth that is not cancerous and does not spread to other parts of the body.

Biopsy: A procedure in which a small sample of tissue is removed and examined under a microscope to check for cancer cells.

Carcinoembryonic Antigen (CEA): A protein often found in higher levels in the blood of people with colorectal cancer. It can be used to monitor cancer recurrence.

Chemotherapy: A type of cancer treatment that uses drugs to kill cancer cells or stop them from growing and dividing.

Colonoscopy: An examination of the colon and rectum using a long, flexible tube with a camera. It's used to screen for colorectal cancer and remove polyps.

Colostomy: A surgical procedure in which an opening (stoma) is created in the abdomen to allow waste to exit the body when part of the colon is removed.

Computed Tomography (CT) Scan: An imaging test that uses X-rays to create detailed cross-sectional images of the body, often used to detect cancer or check for recurrence.

Immunotherapy: A type of cancer treatment that boosts or manipulates the body's immune system to help it fight cancer.

Malignant: A term used to describe a tumor or growth that is cancerous and can invade nearby tissues or spread to other parts of the body.

Metastasis: The spread of cancer cells from the original site to other parts of the body.

Oncologist: A doctor who specializes in diagnosing and treating cancer.

Peripheral Neuropathy: A side effect of some cancer treatments that causes numbness, tingling, or pain in the hands and feet.

Polyp: A small growth on the lining of the colon or rectum. Some polyps can become cancerous over time.

Radiation Therapy: A cancer treatment that uses high-energy radiation to kill cancer cells or shrink tumors.

Recurrence: The return of cancer after treatment and a period of remission.

Resection: A surgical procedure to remove part of an organ or structure, such as a section of the colon or rectum in colorectal cancer treatment.

Staging: A system used to describe the extent of cancer in the body, indicating how advanced the cancer is.

Stoma: An opening created surgically to allow waste to exit the body, often used in colostomies and ileostomies.

Targeted Therapy: A type of cancer treatment that uses drugs designed to specifically target certain molecules in cancer cells, reducing damage to healthy cells.

Tumor: An abnormal mass of tissue that can be benign or malignant (cancerous).

Ultrasound: An imaging test that uses sound waves to create pictures of the inside of the body.

This glossary covers the essential terms related to colorectal cancer and its treatment. Understanding these terms can help you have more informed conversations with your healthcare team and navigate your cancer journey with greater confidence. If you have questions about any of these terms or concepts, don't hesitate to ask your doctor for clarification or further explanation.

List of Helpful Websites and Organizations

American Cancer Society (ACS)

Website: cancer.org
- The ACS provides comprehensive information on all types of cancer, including colorectal cancer. They offer resources on diagnosis, treatment, support services, and survivorship. They also have a 24/7 helpline to answer questions and offer support.

Colorectal Cancer Alliance

Website: ccalliance.org
- This organization is dedicated to supporting individuals with colorectal cancer. It offers patient resources, educational materials, support groups, and information on advocacy and prevention.

CancerCare

Website: cancercare.org
- CancerCare provides free counseling, support groups, educational workshops, and financial assistance for cancer patients. They offer support specifically for those dealing with colorectal cancer.

National Cancer Institute (NCI)

Website: cancer.gov
- The NCI is part of the National Institutes of Health (NIH) and provides extensive information on cancer research, treatment options, clinical trials, and the latest cancer news.

Cancer Support Community

Website: cancersupportcommunity.org
- This organization offers a wide range of support services for cancer patients and their families, including online support groups, educational resources, and a cancer support helpline.

Colorectal Cancer Canada

Website: colorectalcancercanada.com
- Focused on supporting Canadian patients, this organization provides information on colorectal cancer, support groups, patient resources, and advocacy efforts.

LIVESTRONG Foundation

Website: livestrong.org
- LIVESTRONG offers support services for cancer patients, including financial assistance, emotional support, and resources to help navigate life during and after cancer treatment.

Patient Advocate Foundation (PAF)

Website: patientadvocate.org
- PAF provides free case management, patient education, and financial support for cancer patients, including those with colorectal cancer.

ClinicalTrials.gov

Website: clinicaltrials.gov
- This website allows you to search for clinical trials related to colorectal cancer. It's useful for finding research studies and treatment trials that might be relevant to your situation.

These websites and organizations are trusted resources for information, support, and guidance on colorectal cancer. They offer various services, from educational materials and support groups to financial assistance and clinical trials information. If you need additional help or specific resources, these are excellent places to start.

Index

A
- Adjuvant Therapy: Chapter 2 – Treatment Options

- Advance Directives: Chapter 7 – Resources and Support
- American Cancer Society: Chapter 7 – Resources and Support

- Anemia: Chapter 4 – Navigating Treatment

- Anxiety: Chapter 3 – Coping with Diagnosis

B
- Biopsy: Chapter 1 – Understanding Colorectal Cancer

- Blood Tests: Chapter 1 – Understanding Colorectal Cancer

C
- Chemotherapy: Chapter 2 – Treatment Options

- Clinical Trials: Chapter 6 – Clinical Trials and Experimental Treatments

- Colonoscopy: Chapter 1 – Diagnostic Tests and Screening

- Colostomy/Ileostomy: Chapter 4 – Navigating Treatment

- Constipation: Chapter 4 – Navigating Treatment

D

- Diagnosis: Chapter 1 – Understanding Colorectal Cancer

- Diarrhea: Chapter 4 – Navigating Treatment

- Diet and Nutrition: Chapter 4 – Navigating Treatment

E

- Emotional Support: Chapter 3 – Coping with Diagnosis

- Exercise and Physical Activity: Chapter 5 – Living Well with Colorectal Cancer

F

- Fatigue: Chapter 4 – Navigating Treatment

- Family and Medical Leave Act (FMLA): Chapter 7 – Resources and Support

- Financial Assistance: Chapter 7 – Resources and Support

G
- Genetic Testing: Chapter 1 – Diagnostic Tests and Screening
- Glossary: Chapter 8 – Appendices

H
- Health Insurance: Chapter 7 – Resources and Support
- Healthcare Team: Chapter 2 – Treatment Options
- Hope and Encouragement: Chapter 8 – Stories of Hope and Inspiration

I
- Immunotherapy: Chapter 2 – Treatment Options
- Index: Chapter 8 – Appendices
- Informed Consent: Chapter 3 – Coping with Diagnosis
- Diagnosis

L
- Legal Rights: Chapter 7 – Resources and Support
- Lifestyle Changes: Chapter 5 – Living Well with Colorectal Cancer

M
- Managing Side Effects: Chapter 4 – Navigating Treatment
- Mental Well-Being: Chapter 5 – Living Well with Colorectal Cancer

N
- Nutrition and Diet: Chapter 5 – Living Well with Colorectal Cancer

P
- Personal Stories: Chapter 8 – Stories of Hope and Inspiration
- Physical Therapy: Chapter 5 – Recovery and Rehabilitation

R
- Radiation Therapy: Chapter 2 – Treatment Options
- Recurrence: Chapter 5 – Recovery and Rehabilitation

S
- Sexual Health: Chapter 5 – Living Well with Colorectal Cancer
- Side Effects: Chapter 4 – Navigating Treatment
- Surgery: Chapter 2 – Treatment Options

T
- Targeted Therapy: Chapter 2 – Treatment Options

- Transportation Assistance: Chapter 7 – Resources and Support

W
- Workplace Accommodations: Chapter 7 – Resources and Support

Use this index to quickly find information on specific topics throughout this guide. Each topic is linked to the chapter where you can find more detailed explanations and guidance on how to navigate your journey with colorectal cancer.

Note

www.ingramcontent.com/pod-product-compliance
Lightning Source LLC
Chambersburg PA
CBHW071926210526
45479CB00002B/569